Finding
Grace

Finding Grace

AN ALZHEIMER'S TOOLBOX FOR CAREGIVERS, DETAILED IN THE STORY OF ONE WOMAN'S EFFORT TO LOVE HER MOTHER UNTIL THE END

Julie Nielsen

ISBN: 1537322923
ISBN 13: 9781537322926
Library of Congress Control Number: 2016914493
CreateSpace Independent Publishing Platform
North Charleston, South Carolina

Cover photography courtesy of Wei Wang, 2012

Contents

Introduction

wrote this book to educate others on the monumental task that awaits us in determining our own care or the care of people we love. This love requires a fight, and you have to know the rules of the fight—and understand how many people don't play by them. I remember seeing a sign many years ago. It was a takeoff on the Emergency Alert System announcement you hear on the radio. The sign said, "This life is just a test; it is only a test. If this had been a real life, you would have been given further instructions on where to go and what to do." I felt like this a lot, and I asked myself, "How did I get here, and what do I do?"

My mother died on Labor Day 2012, after a long fight with Alzheimer's, but because of the twists and turns of what happened, publication of this book was delayed until 2017. I managed her care for over eight years and learned many valuable lessons along the way. My original goal in writing this book was simply to educate people on some key technology tools that are essential for the protection of cognitively impaired or incapacitated adults as well as on some of the planning concepts and care points I learned by making my own way. But an author-friend pointed out that this would make for a very dry book. So I told our story along the way. Really I told *my* story. Everyone's situation will be different, but I believe every reader will find some commonality.

You should be interested in this topic—out of love for older family members and out of concern for yourself. But data from the Alzheimer's Association's *2017 Alzheimer's Disease Facts and Figures Report* provide additional reasons why we should all be interested.

- As many as 5.5 million people have Alzheimer's, and 200,000 are under the age of sixty-five.
- Every sixty-six seconds someone in the United States develops Alzheimer's; by midcentury it will be every thirty-three seconds.
- Alzheimer's disease is now the sixth-leading cause of death.
- Of the top ten causes of death in the United States, Alzheimer's is the only one that cannot be prevented, cured, or slowed.
- People age 65 and older survive an average of four to eight years after diagnosis, yet some live as long as 20 years with it.
- Over 15 million family and friends provided 18.2 billion hours of informal or unpaid care to those with Alzheimer's and other dementias.
- That care had an estimated economic value of $230.1 billion.

I hope you enjoy reading about my beautiful mother, my love for her, and how anyone's devotion can be put to the test. But most of all, I hope you find tools and tips that you will use and that will improve your life and the lives of those you care for. Because I suspect that if you are reading this book, you are on the journey. I made it, and so will you. I now know where to go and what to do.

Thank you to my friends who didn't forget to remember me during this struggle, and who didn't give up on our friendship. And thanks to the wonderful law enforcement and legal professionals in Fairfax County, Virginia, and at the federal Department of Homeland Security for doing what they do with skill, thoughtfulness, patience, and ingenuity.

Julie Nielsen

You will see in this book that I come from a family of strong women. I learned the importance of caring for each other from my mom, my aunt, and my grandmother. Julie's book demonstrates this value, and gives us the tools we need to care for loved ones as she so selflessly did.

Erica Nielsen
Niece of the author
Granddaughter of Betty Nielsen

Note on Names

The names of the companies I worked with for assisted living and in-home care were changed for the purposes of this book, as were the names of staff associated with them, except for the primary caregiver and her family, upon whom this book's title is based.

CHAPTER 1

History

"One day soon, I'll be one of these faces on the wall."

There were many places I could have started this book. But this statement, which Mom made as we stood in her condo, hanging pictures, starts the story best. Her words were sad, but they encouraged me too. I changed the subject that day, as it was easy to do, but the words stuck. Almost every day, I now think about what I'll do before I am one of those faces on a wall.

The story starts there, but to fully understand, I need to go back further. Let me introduce myself. I was born in 1964 (which made me forty-nine when I started writing this book), the daughter of a teacher and a naval officer, and the sister of one older brother, Chris, whom I idolized ever since I could say his name. Mom and Dad both came from broken homes, but Dad's was worse. As I understand it, his father was the classic Depression-era dad who went out for a loaf of bread and never came back. I didn't know this man, other than from a fireplace toolset and a hallway table he made by hand, both of which now sit in my home. But he was still a part of my life in that he lived in my brain as an example of the things we were not. He was someone who ran when it got tough. We were quite the opposite.

Dad's mom was always old to me—Grandma, quiet and graceful. In her working years, she cleaned houses and took in ironing to provide for her two sons. They lived in poverty and survived with the help of the church. Dad used to say that they were the homeless of today—living on the edge but for the grace of strangers. Later she owned a home, a small house with a rock foundation and a big garage full of surprises.

Dad's brother, Uncle Bob, lived with her and died when I was five. He was a young man plagued by epilepsy and, as my dad would find out later, heart trouble. I was too young to fully appreciate Grandma. She stayed in Minnesota, where Dad was from. We traveled there periodically, and she visited us. And since it was Minnesota, we went there in the warm weather, swimming in lakes and getting bitten by mosquitos so big that I swore at the time they could have flown away with me. Grandma developed some sort of dementia when I was in elementary school and died when I was in junior high. When she died, it was winter. The deep Minnesota snow and ice surprised me, and I remember shades of gray when I think about that last trip. Based on what my dad was like, Grandma must have been a strong and beautiful woman.

Mom lived in near poverty too, but it was different. Her parents divorced when she was young, but both her mother and father were active in her life. She adored them both, and they all struggled financially. Mom lived with her mother, whom I knew as Grandbill. Her name was Willie, nicknamed Billie, and later Grandbill to her two grandkids. Both parents worked long hours, and Mom was an early "latchkey kid." They too were also early homeless, at times living with Grandbill's sister and her daughters, whom I know as Mom's sisters instead of her cousins. Mom's dad later remarried and died of Parkinson's before I was born, I think around 1959. He lives in my memory as "Daddy." When Mom was in college, Grandbill remarried a man named Richard Killough, the man I know as Grandpa. As an example of my mother's early fortitude, she confronted the man who would become her stepfather and demanded that he either leave or stop drinking immediately. My mother had seen the signs of alcoholism and was a fierce protector of her mother. He stopped and, as far as I know, died many years later without ever drinking another drop.

Mom and Dad did all of their moving with the navy before I was born. By the time I came along in Norfolk, Virginia, they had been in Vietnam, Albuquerque, and other places. Before I was a year old, we settled in the Washington, DC, suburbs in northern Virginia. We were close to Grandbill and Grandpa. Almost every Christmas we piled in the station wagon and drove to Memphis, where they lived. We talked frequently by phone (back when that was an expensive thing to do), and they are still a vivid part of my childhood and my memory. In their later years, they moved to Virginia to be near us so we could care for them. Grandpa died when I was a freshman in college, and Grandbill when I was a sophomore. It makes me sad now that I wasn't there to support my mom as her mother and stepfather died. I would have been better prepared for what was to come. But I saw enough to know the unwavering faithfulness Mom had to them.

Our family was a great example of the fact that you could come from a broken home and still get it right when you have your own family. Both Mom and Dad made it to college. Dad headed for the navy and went off to see the world beyond Minneapolis. Mom headed for California after going to school in Waco, Texas, and discovered military men (and my dad) in Long Beach, California. My parents were the essence of proper parenting—not too strict, not too lenient, not too indulgent, and incredibly loving. They wanted their kids to have what they did not. And while most of their lives revolved around raising us, they were good at making time for dates and time together. Their marriage was strong. As we grew up, we saw families stumble and break. But ours held firm. I remember being terrified on the few occasions where my parents would argue. Surely that must mean they could divorce, as I saw with parents of friends. Later, when I shared that with my mother, she was horrified. And I've since learned that some healthy arguing can be good.

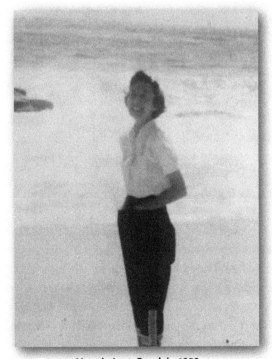

Mom in Long Beach in 1958

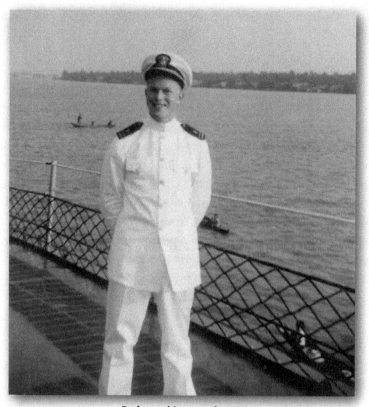

Dad on a ship around 1958

At four years apart, Chris and I bickered—a lot. In fact, I remember one morning Mom said, "You two make me want to just run away from home."

"Who would make my breakfast?" I asked selfishly.

But Chris and I played and grew up together. When he was a teen, I had crushes on his friends. It wasn't until my first date that I realized Chris actually cared about me. "Who is he?" he asked. And he stayed home that night so he could meet the unsuspecting boy. "Oh, and wear that fuzzy sweater...guys like those. On second thought, don't." I look back on this so fondly. I suspect my brother was my protector long before I knew it. He would be my protector as we moved into adulthood too—the one I would call to do the heavy lifting and to get advice on just about anything. If he didn't know, he would figure it out.

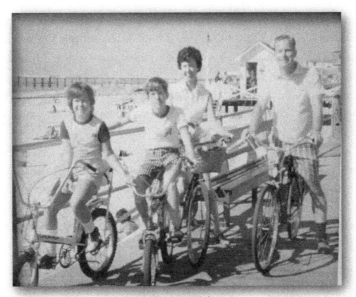

The late-1960s Nielsens

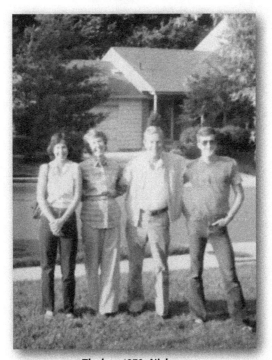

The late-1970s Nielsens

Chris went into law enforcement, first as a beat police officer in Fairfax County, Virginia, and later as a detective in Roanoke County, Virginia. I went the business route, getting an undergraduate degree in business at Auburn University and later a graduate degree from Marymount University back in DC. I landed in the human resource field immediately and found my niche. I had my mom's gift of gab and an outgoing personality, and as a result I dated a lot, but I never married. I love what I do, and I suppose I married my career.

After I graduated from college, Mom and Dad retired to Carlsbad, California, a little north of San Diego. They chose a home carefully, making sure it was small enough for Mom to handle if something happened to Dad. They loved the weather, the gardening, and the traveling—everything. They made retirement what we would all like it to be.

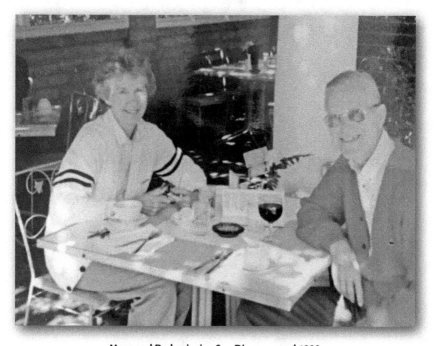

Mom and Dad enjoying San Diego around 1988

After losing their first baby, Chris and his wife got pregnant again fairly quickly. My niece, Erica, was born in 1991. We all spent the following Christmas together, and it was a beautiful time. Then, on January 7, I got the phone call from Chris while I was at work: Dad was dead. It was as though a bomb went off in my life. I wasn't married. Dad hadn't given me away yet. "I'll give you away," Chris said at the airport when we both arrived in San Diego late that night. "I've always wanted to give you away!" We laughed through tears. Life was not supposed to happen this way. Dad's health hadn't been good, and we knew his heart wouldn't let him live to be very old. But we didn't expect it at fifty-nine.

There had been an earlier, smaller bomb. I was too young to recognize its explosive danger and how it would later reach into my life. Dad had his first heart attack at forty. He'd been in the hospital for tests, and because he was being monitored, the alarms went off right away. Code Blue at Fairfax Hospital. A call in the middle of the night. I didn't get the gravity of the words Mom heard: "You'd better come and bring your kids. We don't think your husband is going to make it." I was clueless at the hospital. I remember being afraid of what I might see, and I didn't go into Dad's room in the ICU. It still nags at me today. What if that had been it and I was too afraid to say good-bye? Dad recovered, but he struggled with heart health until the day I was the one getting that call.

At the funeral, twenty-one guns saluted my father, and the sound of each round made me jump. They didn't play "Taps"; Mom asked them not to, since it had always made her sad. Dad was cremated and buried in a military cemetery in San Diego. I'm not sure how much I mourned the loss of the greatest man I ever knew. I was shattered, but I had to take care of my mom, and that drove everything. I put Mom ahead of myself, as I had seen her do with her mom, and pushed ahead. The finances, the funeral, the aftermath—all were a blur. Chris took care of the financial arrangements, and I became my mother's right hand and confidante, in addition to already being her best friend (and she, mine). Mom was already heavily involved in the finances, and that would continue for years. We had talked frequently even before Dad died, but after his death, it was an unusual night that we didn't talk to at least say good night. Even without Dad, I knew we had something special.

It seems odd to me now, but despite having such a close family, we didn't grow up saying "I love you." Don't get me wrong. We loved each other a lot. We just didn't *say* it. But on the day Dad died, as I hung up the phone from that awful conversation with Chris, we said, "I love you." And then, as I called my mother through tears, I said it again. Just about every conversation ended that way from that day on.

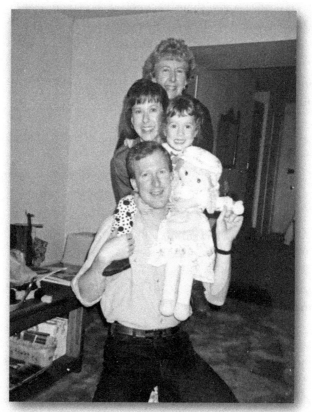

Mom, Chris, Erica, and me playing in my living room on one of Mom's early trips east

And so it went. Chris and his wife had another child, my nephew, Rick, in 1996. Mom made many trips to Virginia. I made many trips to California. Chris raised his family, and I worked and dated. The laughter when we all got together was wonderful. I can make myself laugh now thinking about us all at the dinner table.

CHAPTER 2

The Call

On one of Mom's early trips to Virginia, we stopped for lunch at a café, the kind where you stand up and order and take your food to a table. Mom was in front of me. Behind me was a lovely elderly woman. I smiled at her and said hello, as I typically did. I had always been in tune with the elderly, and seeing them alone touched my heart even when I was a child. A voice from behind her was harsh. "*Mom!* Will you just pick something!" exclaimed a woman. She was angry and in a hurry. Her mother studied her options, moving painfully slowly. "Can't you just make up your mind?" the daughter asked. It hurt to hear her frustration. I can picture them to this day. I made a mental note that I could never, would never, become like the daughter.
~~that~~

I don't know exactly what "normal" old age is supposed to look like. I noticed things changing in my mom. Minor forgetfulness. The woman who was in charge of the checkbook for decades began to have trouble balancing one. Sometimes I would help over the phone. At other times she would save statements, and we'd go through them painstakingly when she came east or I went west. She never liked my idea of simply trusting the bank and acknowledging that they rarely made mistakes.

I would broach the subject of her moving to Virginia, but she loved her beautiful little house in Carlsbad and didn't want to leave. "I'll come back when I need to," she would say. I knew she would too, and I wasn't overly worried about the timing. And then one Tuesday night, my phone rang. Our old family friend Margaret, who, with her husband, had followed Mom and Dad to Carlsbad, called in tears and with a shaking voice. I remember it clearly. "I've been putting off this call…I didn't want to make it," she said. "I've spent time with my pastor trying to make sure I do it right. Something is wrong with your mom, and you don't see it. We think it's Alzheimer's." According to Margaret, Mom had been locking her keys in the car, making lunch appointments and then forgetting them, and doing some other unusual things.

Another bomb. This could not happen to me. It was supposed to happen to other people. How could my mom get Alzheimer's? A doctor wouldn't say that word for a few months, but I knew. How could I lose my father *and* my mother this young? I was shattered again. I was on my knees when I called Chris. I could hear the tears in his voice—Margaret had called him first, and he was waiting for my call. We got ourselves together. It was a couple of weeks before Mother's Day, and we decided my gift to Mom would be a visit from me.

I spoke to our long-time friend Annie the next day. "Bert," she said, "you're going to have to put on your big-girl panties and get this done." Bert was short for Bertina, the nickname she'd assigned to me at birth because I was born on her dog's birthday. I was Little Bertie Wooster's namesake. If I had a godmother, Annie would be it. She likes to call herself "Bert's other mother." She was planning a drive up from Virginia Beach to tell me in person that she too was seeing problems with Mom, but Margaret had beaten her to it. She would be one of those consistent voices over the coming years, saying, "Take time for yourself," and, "You know I'm here." But above all it was, "You can do this." She was always my kick in the butt when I needed it. Annie had taken care of her mother too, and she knew exactly where I was. And where I was headed.

The Missing Checkbook

The trip was uneventful. Nothing happened to make me panic. But for the first time, I could tell my mom was acting. She would talk as though she knew something, but there was nothing underneath. Still, we got out and had a good time. We ate out as we loved to do and visited friends, and this time I pushed harder at the idea of moving. "Absolutely not," Mom replied. I was scheduled to fly home Monday, and when I went into the office-bedroom to get something, I saw a pack of starter checks on the desk. I stared at them for a moment and pondered what they could be from. Mom had let me take over her finances a year before, and I was paying her bills. Her income went into one account, and I paid all of the expenses from it.

"Mom, what are these checks from?" I called out.

"Oh, I lost my checkbook and had to open a new account."

"Oh no...you can't *do* that, Mom! When? How? Oh God...where is the money?"

Mom looked a little confused at my shock. We left the suitcase and charged out the door to the bank. They had indeed closed the master account. "No," they said, "once it's closed, there is nothing that can be done to reopen it." And then, "No, there is nothing that can be done to prevent it in the future." If Mom's name was on the account, she could do whatever she wanted. At least the manager at the bank had a good idea: create a small account for Mom to know about, and let me use the bigger account. If she lost the checkbook, only a small amount of money would be at risk. I felt sick as we left the bank, and I felt an ominous cloud overhead. Things were starting to happen, and I was normally three thousand miles away. This wasn't going to work.

The bank-account incident was my first experience of dealing with the government as I tried to redirect deposits into the new accounts. And it turned out that the checkbook was never really lost. Mom had developed a tendency to think things were lost when they weren't.

From the airport a day later, I called Mom's doctor. He was a gruff and, I thought, somewhat rude man. He couldn't say much to me because Mom had not authorized it, but he made a huge exception. In an impatient outburst, he said, "Ms. Nielsen, your mother has Alzheimer's. You need to move her to Virginia now while she still knows what's going on, or else she'll wake up in a strange place every day for the rest of her life." Then he said something critical that everyone dealing with Alzheimer's needs to know: "You need to move fast so that wherever you put your mother is in her long-term memory, not her short-term memory." This turned out to be great advice, because Mom's long-term memory was good for a long time. But the things that had just happened or just been discussed seemed to fall out of her brain immediately.

Care Concept #1: Make Decisions and Moves Early to Keep "Home" in Long-Term Memory

Eventually, Alzheimer's will steal both short-term and long-term memory. But in the beginning, and possibly for a long time, it will steal only the short-term.

This is why people with the disease repeat themselves as though conversations from five minutes ago didn't happen. As soon as it's clear there is some sort of dementia—Alzheimer's or some other type—make decisions fast, and move toward the future, whatever it is. Better yet, make those decisions when there are no problems. Waiting to move to assisted living until someone is in bad shape is, well, mean. It is like forcing them to live out the movie *Groundhog Day*. They could wake up every morning not knowing where they are because they forgot. Again. Alternatively, waiting too long to move a person's caregiver into the home means there will always be a stranger in the house, not a known and remembered face.

Do you sometimes feel like you are watching your life on television? I do a lot. Travelers were hustling around me as I stood at my gate. Why were they all acting like nothing was wrong? Back in Virginia, Chris and I talked late that night, discussing whether we should tell Mom she had Alzheimer's. He leaned toward yes, and I leaned toward no.

"Wouldn't you want to know?" he asked.

"At my age now, yes. But what does it get Mom at her age?" I responded. Mom was happy, and to me, this sounded like the most depressing news I could imagine. And I knew it was her worst nightmare. Ultimately, Chris deferred to me. My mother would never know.

How Do You Write a Check?

One night, Mom needed to write a check for something. As we talked, it became clear that she had forgotten how to do this basic task. I was a little impatient at first, and I remembered the café woman. And then I realized how clueless Mom really was. How could she just forget how to write a check? I asked Mom if she could hold on for just a minute while I dialed Chris's number and prayed he would answer the phone. I just had time to say, "Just listen. Mom doesn't know you're on." The flash button reconnected Mom and me, and we went through the painful details of writing a check, and I had her read it back to me. After we hung up, I called Chris back, and all I could say was, "Oh God..." He had been researching dementia online as he listened, and he read the key facts to me. He read the road map of where our lives would ultimately go. Alzheimer's is only one kind of dementia. Doctors say no one knows for sure if it's Alzheimer's until an autopsy. But the dementia was a given.

We already had a ticket for Mom to come to Virginia two weeks later for her annual spring trip. So that was our plan. We had our normal fun. Chris and the kids came up. Lots of laughter. Mom was an avid driver. As usual with Mom's trips, I would find other transportation to work, and she would keep my car. That Thursday night, we filled the tank with gas. I had gotten Mom a cell phone by then—the simplest one I could find, with instructions taped on the back. I reminded her how to use the phone as I left for work Friday. That night after work on the way to dinner, I looked at the gas gauge. "Mom, why does it look like the gas tank is less than half full?" Mom was irritated and told me not to make a big deal of it. Then out came her story of the day. She had dropped me off and taken a wrong turn. She described landmarks she had seen. I identified her path as she talked, recognizing landmarks in DC, Maryland, and western Fairfax County in Virginia. Until now I hadn't worried about Mom's driving. I had been raised here, and Mom still knew her way around. But somehow that knowledge seemed to have left her. "Why didn't you call me?" I asked. "I would have come and found you!" She was completely unable to grasp the cell-phone concept. The cloud was there again. Things were changing.

I contemplated moving Mom in with me, but I sensed early on that this would be a long haul. I had a three-story townhouse, and the stairs were steep. Mom handled them well on visits, but that wouldn't last for long. I also knew that I would eventually need a safe haven for myself. Mom was nowhere near ready for assisted living. "That's for old people," she would say. A move to assisted living would trigger the beginning of the depletion of Mom's resources. And I knew the general costs already. The thought of moving us both to a house without stairs never seemed very practical. So I kept the move-in option as my worst-case scenario—the nuclear option that would mean everything had collapsed.

An important thing happened on this trip. On the last day, as I tried to determine our next steps, I suggested we go look at the apartments up the street from me. Mom was clearly not impressed and could see I had a game plan. "No," she said flatly.

"Please?" I implored.

"Okay. Fine. We'll go look. But I'm not moving."

I called ahead and talked to the property manager. Yes, he would pretend there was a waiting list. He must have thought the situation was rather odd. This was my first, as someone else would term it later, "elder fib." My parents had raised Chris and me to tell the truth, however painful. I was the kid who took it to the extreme, always telling my parents when I had done something wrong. Chris was a little more lax when it came to that rule. But I would learn that elder fibs were required to protect my mother.

>>> **Care Point 1** <<<
Elder fibs aren't lies. Use them to gently push people in the right direction.

The Renaissance was beautiful. Mom and I both saw the attraction of living in a pretty building where everything was taken care of for you. Before we left, we met with the property manager and carefully described what she was looking for. Sixth floor, because Mom had read years ago that the fire department couldn't get past seven, and she didn't want to push it. I wanted a certain side of the building, away from Washington's busy Beltway. And a two-bedroom so Mom could have company. The manager dutifully noted what we wanted and gave me a knowing look. "Mrs. Nielsen, I'll let you know when something like this opens up."

Mom smiled at him sweetly and said, "Thank you, but I'm not moving. My daughter is making this up." However, she also said she liked what she'd seen. And she wasn't looking at me like she wanted to kill me anymore. Progress. Mom flew home to California the next day.

The Good, the Bad, the Mean, and the Dumb

Throughout the time I spent with my mom over these years, I came across good people and bad people, helpful people and mean people, smart people and dumb people. And I came to depend on the good, helpful, and smart ones. I suffered through the bad, mean, and dumb ones. Perhaps they were simply ignorant. Never was that clearer than the stage where I was ramping up my efforts to get her moved. I was noticing more issues now. Mom was seeing a second doctor, and I decided to call and see if they could be of any help. The helpful nurse turned cross as she realized she was in danger of violating HIPPA laws. I remained nice and thanked her—and asked her not to tell Mom I had called.

That night, Mom called and said that the nurse had told her I called. I was stunned. They didn't have to talk to me. But did they have to tell her I called? Was it not clear we were a mother and daughter in crisis? They couldn't have just said, "No, we can't help you"? I took a deep breath. Mom seemed nonplussed by it, which was another sign of the disease. My real mom would have been furious. Crisis averted. But a week later, I had another idea. She was back at the same doctor. I called to see if they could have her sign a release while she was there. The answer was a harsh no, but it was the words that came after that caused me to come unglued—a rare rage for me. The nurse said, "Something is very wrong. Your mother was so confused when she was here today that I had to walk her to her car." It was the same woman who thought it was acceptable to tell my fiercely independent mother I was trying to intervene.

It was late in the evening on the East Coast, and few of my coworkers were still around. It was as though someone had struck a match and lit my fuse. I exploded. "My mother was confused, and you let her get in her car? You put her in her car? What was wrong? Where is she?" I was furious. I could tell, from three thousand miles away, that I had hit my mark. The nurse panicked as she realized what she'd done. "You'd better hope I find my mother," was all I could think to say as I hung up. I hoped the woman was frightened. HIPPA was nothing compared to what I could do if my mom was really missing. I felt painfully helpless as I contemplated the miles and made flight reservations, which would not get me to California for hours.

Mom's neighbors were angelic. Everyone had moved to the neighborhood at the same time back in 1987 or so. Mom and Dad were the grandparents of the neighborhood and had been surrounded by young families just starting out. They had participated in Fourth of July cookouts, Christmas caroling, and summer shows produced by the kids. It was a wonderful place to raise a family and a wonderful place for my parents to grow old. The neighbors had always kept an eye out, especially after Dad died. I had visited with them during that Mother's Day trip and was in contact with them, so their vigilance had increased. On this day, I called the neighbors who lived closest to Mom for help. But after just a few minutes, my phone rang. Mom had pulled into the driveway, waving, and they all rushed out to meet her. The drive home from San Diego was stuck in her long-term memory.

The good news was that she was back. The bad news was that it was obvious something was wrong with her. Everyone could see the indicators, but what could have changed so dramatically overnight? Michelle, our neighbor on one side, was a nurse, and she strolled into the house with Mom. She went through Mom's medicines with her. There she found the problem: Mom had somehow switched her heart medicine with her thyroid medicine. Not only was the switch the cause of Mom's sudden terrible confusion, but the combination was deadly and could have killed her. Michelle went out and purchased dispensers for the time being, and she loaded them up for the week. She took all of Mom's meds with her as she left. Mom returned to her normal state. The crisis was averted for now.

>>> Care Point 2 <<<
People with dementia are good actors—which means they are in more danger than you think.

That night, I sat at the computer looking at page after page of medicine dispensers. And there it was: the Philips Medication Dispenser (at the time it was called MD2). It was a computerized dispenser that looked like a large coffeepot and was meant to be loaded by a family member or caregiver. (It looks more modern now, is mobile, and the options have changed.) Within minutes I eagerly plunked down about $700, and PMD was headed for Virginia so I could figure him out.

It wasn't that hard. PMD needed electricity, a phone line (now a smartphone), and someone to load meds in little plastic cups and then load the cups into it. It seemed simple enough. I called Craig and Leslie, neighbors on the other side, and asked if they'd be willing to help until I could get Mom moved. They were game, so off PMD went to his new life in California, with the first month of medicine cups ready to go. For several months, I would fill the cups in Virginia and ship them to Craig, and he would walk next door to load them.

That description sounds a little easier than it actually was, though. Mom hated PMD. He sat in the kitchen and took up a chunk of counter space. Worse yet, people could see him, and "she did not need help from me or any of the neighbors." The first night after Craig set PMD up, Mom and I had the worst argument I ever remember us having. It was awful, and I called Chris in tears. I couldn't move fast enough to keep her safe. Mom was furious. I didn't know what to do. I never did learn what Chris said to her, but Mom acquiesced, and PMD continued to live on the counter. He would call out, "It's *time* to take your medicine" at the appropriate dispensing times. And then if Mom didn't push the button after an hour, PMD would call his "real" home in New Jersey, and the people at the monitoring station would call me. Mom never quite figured that part out. But when he would call out, Mom would say, "Oh shit." For a few weeks, we called him Dr. Ohshit. But as he became a part of our lives, I pointed out that this wasn't entirely appropriate, since we sometimes talked about him in public. So PMD became known as Dr. Ohno for the rest of his life with us.

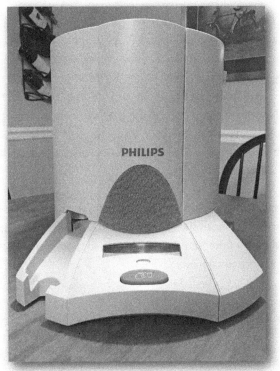

A later version of "Dr. Ohno." He was an essential part of our lives and would help keep Mom out of assisted living for two years. The device is now called the Philips Medication Dispenser (PMD) and is sold by Phillips. We would have run out of money without him.

Let's stop here and talk about Dr. Ohno. PMD is more than a medicine dispenser. It also provided fall or illness protection for Mom. For example, he was scheduled to tell Mom at 8:00 a.m. that it was time for her morning meds. He would call repeatedly, getting louder and louder, and more irritating. At 9:00 a.m., barring the required push of his big red button, he would send out an alert. Then I would get a warning call. It was rare for us. But I knew that if Mom were to fall during the night, the absolute worst case was that she'd be on the floor until 9:00 a.m. By then I'd have gotten a call and would have been on the phone to the neighbors or, once she moved to Virginia, headed to her home to see what was wrong. That particular scenario never happened, but it could have, and I was ready. PMD was my extra set of eyes. He was programmed to report in on a daily basis to ensure that communication problems didn't cause the system to crash.

PMD has a bigger benefit with national implications. When all was said and done, it kept Mom out of assisted living for over two years. Many American seniors end up in assisted living—on their own dime or on the dime of taxpayers—because of the inability to take meds, to the tune of $5,000 to $8,000 per month. Let's use $6,500 as a sample national estimate. That's $78,000 per year. We were at the higher end because of our location. Looking back now, I see that without PMD, one of my worst fears would have come true: we would have run out of money. And at the rate I was going, my worst fears had a habit of coming true.

There is one weakness to PMD. Just because someone presses the button and picks up the cup doesn't mean she is going to actually take the meds. But in my experience, it worked most of the time. When Mom held the meds in her hand, it allowed her long-term memory to take over.

Technology Tool #1: Philips Medication Dispenser (PMD)

PMD does an excellent job of dispensing the right meds at the right time. If you are local, you can easily run PMD for your loved one. If you are not local, you can still manage the meds with the loading help of a friend or neighbor. PMD also provides an extra communication layer. Failure to push the dispensing button could signal other trouble—like a fall. It can also serve as a reminder for meds such as liquids that are not dispensed by the system. The unit can be purchased or leased now.

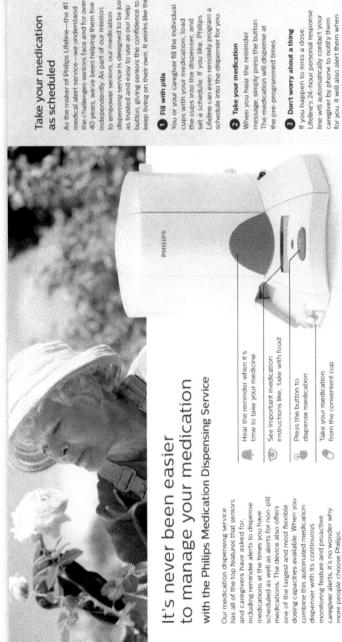

It's never been easier to manage your medication

with the Philips Medication Dispensing Service

Our medication dispensing service has all of the top features that seniors and caregivers have asked for, including reminder alerts to dispense medications at the times you have scheduled as well as alerts for non-pill medications. The device also offers one of the largest and most flexible dosing capacities available. When you combine this automated medication dispenser with its continuous monitoring feature and proactive caregiver alerts, it's no wonder why more people choose Philips.

- Hear the reminder when it's time to take your medicine
- See important medication instructions like, 'take with food'
- Press the button to dispense medication
- Take your medication from the convenient cup

Philips Medication Dispensing Service gives you peace of mind to enjoy life.

Call 1-800-Lifeline for more information or to order.

Take your medication as scheduled

As the maker of Philips Lifeline—the #1 medical alert service—we understand the challenges seniors face and for over 40 years, we've been helping them live independently. As part of our mission to empower seniors, our medication dispensing service is designed to be just as trusted and easy to use as our help button, giving seniors the confidence to keep living on their own. It works like this:

1 Fill with pills
You or your caregiver fill the individual cups with your medication, load the cups into the dispenser, and set a schedule. If you like, Philips Lifeline can even remotely program a schedule into the dispenser for you.

2 Take your medication
When you hear the reminder message, simply press the button. The medication will dispense at the pre-programmed times.

3 Don't worry about a thing
If you happen to miss a dose, Lifeline's 24-hour personal response line will automatically contact your caregiver by phone to notify them for you. It will also alert them when it's time to refill your medications.

Photo courtesy of Philips

Technology is transforming caregiving. Keep an eye on the constant changes and new tools. The company e-pill now has another medication-dispensing option as well.

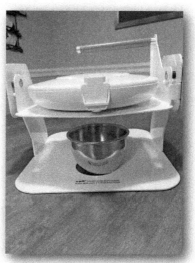

Another medicine-dispensing option on the market now, sold by e-pill (epill. com). But Mom needed one she couldn't pick up and throw away!

CHAPTER 3

The Move

t was late June and time for "the call." On cue, the manager at the Renaissance called Mom and told her that the ideal unit had just become available—sixth floor, the quiet side, and a beautiful balcony. That night I called Mom to tell her I too had gotten a call from them, as though I was surprised. "No, Julie—I'm not moving," she insisted. I was ready for battle. But oddly, it didn't come as I expected.

"It's the perfect unit, Mom, and it could be years before another perfect one opens up. We can't let it go," I said.

"No," she responded.

I wasn't deterred. Failure wasn't an option. The next day, I signed the lease with a move-in date in August. Then I called Mom again that night.

I think three things contributed to what happened next. One was the disease again—Mom was unsure of herself and more willing for me to take the lead. Next was the fact that I played on her natural mothering tendencies. I cried. "This isn't just about you, Mom," I said. "It's my life too, and right now it's a mess." My parents always put their kids first, and I called on that trait for support. And as Mom wavered, I said flatly, "If you move near me, I'll take you to the Ritz Carlton for breakfast once a week."

Mom sounded irritated as she sighed and said, "Oh, okay." I think she knew she had to go. She also loved eating breakfast out. That part was easier than I expected.

I was elated when I called Chris. We decided that I would get her moved, and he would sell the house. The economy in southern California was weakening, and housing prices were declining. We didn't know it, but they were about to take a major tumble. This was a big deal because a lot of the money we would depend on in Virginia was wrapped up in a beautiful little house in California.

It's probably good that I went into human resource management as a career. Project management skills are a must. So I approached the move the way I approached my job. What was the goal? What about the timing and the constraints? And I planned.

I left Washington on a hot August Friday evening, knowing that when I came back, life would be very different. At every turn, I knew I was facing a "last time." The last time Mom would meet me at the San Diego airport. That last drive to her house. The last meal at our favorite restaurants. But there was no time for sadness. I was a woman on a mission. I went over the plan with Mom that night, breaking down the house room by room and spelling out what had to be done each day before we went to bed. The packers were coming Thursday, the movers on Friday, and the cleaners on Saturday. Saturday would be our day to visit with neighbors as well. Sunday we would board a plane and be on our way east.

Care Concept #2: Document and Share

For people with Alzheimer's, what's foreign is scary. And just about everything new is foreign. When making big changes—such as a move—have a plan and share it. Especially with people in the early stages of dementia, share the details, write notes, and include them in the action. The known is much safer than the unknown.

It worked. We plowed through each room as planned. It was easy to get rid of some things, but hard to get rid of others. I had the floor map of the condo with me and would stop and measure what would fit. The donation pile in the garage grew and grew until the car had to stay in the driveway. This first downsizing was hard, and we moved things to Virginia that we shouldn't have. But we probably did pretty well. The apartment was large and would eventually hold all things deemed special.

We mixed in errands, like the bank and the vet. We had to get Mom's aging cat, TC, ready for flight. TC was the cat Mom was not going to have. We had owned only dogs when I was growing up. I had laughed when she started feeding the hungry cat in her backyard, knowing that she wouldn't be able to hold out for long. She would ask at doctors' offices and grocery stores, "Would you like a nice cat?" It wasn't long before she told me one night that "the cat" was so cute sleeping on her couch. She was hooked. I was glad she had company. He became TC, short for "the cat." We are a pet family, and I had been through enough to know by the time of the move that TC wasn't long for this world. But with the vet's blessing, we prepared him for the move. I held my breath the following Saturday evening when he slyly slipped out the front door. He tolerated only my mother, but I sighed in relief when I was able to get my hands around him and carry him to safety. That was one crisis we didn't need.

Thursday came. Packers and movers are really salt-of-the-earth people, and they treated us with great care. They could see what was happening: a life unwillingly getting packed into boxes. Working side by side, we talked about our lives. We all had struggles. One was having major car trouble, and his family was clearly struggling financially. I had already put the better of Mom's two cars on a transport truck headed east, where it would be waiting for her when she arrived. But the other one, an aging Oldsmobile that she and Dad had bought, was still in the driveway. "Would you like our other car?" I asked him. He said yes but admitted he couldn't afford much of anything. I said, "Come back Saturday morning, and get the car that we aren't moving to Virginia. For free." I didn't have time to sell it and was planning on donating it. Mom grinned and loved this opportunity to help someone. That night we still had beds and fell into them, exhausted.

The car thing was an ongoing joke. Why did an elderly woman who didn't go many places need two cars? But after Dad died, no one could persuade Mom to get rid of one. Maybe it was the trips she and Dad had taken in it. No arguments about insurance and maintenance costs could sway her. She liked having a backup. "What if I have car trouble?" she'd ask.

"Taxi?" I would answer.

That argument wasn't won until the move, and even then it was because she knew my car would play backup in Virginia. I inherited Mom's planning ability, and having a "backup to the backup" would serve me well over the coming years. I learned to have a plan and be flexible about changing it.

Friday morning came. I heard the rumble of a truck. There was something moving about what I saw (and I don't mean because it was a "moving truck"). In huge letters across the top of the van it said "Washington, DC." It seemed very fitting that our truck would be based in DC—we were headed home. In hours, all the boxes and furniture were on a truck, and more salt-of-the-earth people were wishing us well. In a stroke of luck, the driver was headed home with no contents other than ours—a cross-country run with only rest stops. "I'll see you next week," he said as we shook hands in front of the house. And off the truck rumbled. The empty house no longer felt like home. The neighbors had loaned us chairs and air mattresses for our last two nights. It was sparse, to say the least.

Friday night, my phone rang. It was PMD's people, worried because he hadn't checked in. I apologized for not warning them that he was disconnected for a little while. We got a good laugh out of Dr. Ohno being trapped in a box, where Mom hoped he would stay. Secretly, I already had a place picked out for him.

Saturday was filled with good-byes. The neighborhood turned out for a big cook-out in Mom's honor. The packer came back, and it felt good to drop the keys in his hand and watch him drive off in my parents' car.

On Sunday, we all acted happy and as though things were normal as Margaret drove us to breakfast and then to the airport. On the plane, Mom and I laughed at me pretending I had a cough every time TC would wail from under my seat. I was proud of myself and what I had accomplished in a week. I leaned my head back and was optimistic as the plane took off and headed east.

CHAPTER 4

The Arrival

What happened after landing was as bad as the move was good. Everything had gone as planned with the move. It was challenging but smooth. Friends raved about the job I did. Chris was impressed. And then the challenge of living with an aging parent with dementia kicked in and ran over me like a runaway train. I never saw it coming.

The moving company showed up as planned. Chris drove up, and in a weekend, we converted the apartment into Mom's Carlsbad home. Furniture arrangements and picture arrangements were as close to the original as possible. In the mornings, sunshine streamed in to the entire condo. Later we would find a beautiful view of fall foliage from the balcony, and then snowcapped trees in the winter.

No one ever told me that a big company like Verizon could not get phone service up and running for a month. Begging and playing on their sympathy did nothing to fix the situation. Mom was still hopelessly (and permanently) afraid of the cell phone, and I was afraid to leave her there without any way to call for help. So Mom stayed with me. The good thing about that was the bird's-eye view I got of Mom's mental state. The bad thing was the acceleration of the role reversal. I'd call from work to make sure things were okay, get home, cook or help cook dinner, and try to finish working at night without Mom knowing. "You're working too hard and running too fast," was her common refrain. But she wanted, and I felt like I owed her, more attention. I was the one who'd said she had to move. My CEO, Tony, had been very patient with my newly added role as caregiver. But I was a senior leader at a well-known organization and had a big role to play.

Finally, the day came, and we moved Mom into her condo. She adapted relatively quickly, again because of the disease—it seemed to dull what would have otherwise been traumatic. I had a heart-stopping moment when she appeared to not be able to find her unit when coming in from the outside. That could kill the whole thing. But after a few ins and outs, she got the hang of it. I remembered the words of the doctor: "You need to move her to Virginia now while she still knows what's going on, or else she'll wake up in a strange place for the rest of her life." We quickly established good relationships with the security guards—more salt-of-the-earth people. I knew they were the people who would see my mom on camera if she ever tried to leave. I never said it, but I observed all of the camera locations and areas of danger. My number would eventually be taped to the main desk in case of emergency, and it was used many times over the years.

Dr. Ohno took up his position in the bedroom and resumed his integral role in our lives. He was in place when Mom first stepped in to see her beautiful apartment, and she never blinked. Loyal friends Barbara and John and Ruth and Keith—couples who were friends of the family since before I was born—stepped in to help. They went to lunch and movies. They sat and laughed and talked about old times. They demonstrated the true friendships that we all hope to have—friendships that had survived good times and bad. Friends who were in it till the end. As hard as it was for me to see my mom with this disease, I knew it was hard on them too. They must have all been in their early thirties when they met. And their deep commitment to Mom spilled over to me.

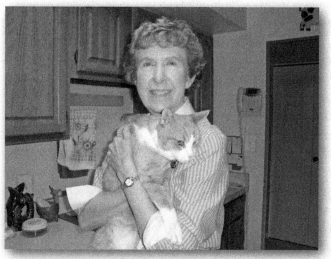

Mom and TC in the kitchen of her condo on move-in day

I was Mom's social secretary and primary entertainer. And after all, I had asked for this, right? But my planning had stopped short of the finish line. It never dawned on me to plan for the next phase.

Chris was always available to back me up, but more for the big things. If I needed him any time of day, I knew he'd be in his car and on the highway in no time. His way of saying "I love you" was to do something for you. On one visit down to Salem, he spent hours detailing my car. It looked brand new by the time he was done. We both beamed, he because he had done something big for me, and I because I knew my brother loved me. But he was almost four hours away and was very involved with his kids, so I was the default caregiver.

The Biggest Missed Opportunity

On a Saturday morning, I drove to our insurance agent's office. "Talk to me about long-term care," I said to Eric.

"We can set you up, but get ready for the price tag," he said. And then he laid it on me: $20,000 a year, at least.

"Twenty thousand," I repeated, letting it sink in. That sounded like a lot of money at the time, and it was. But later, we would be running through over $8,000 a month, making the $20,000 look like a drop in the bucket. I didn't know much about this at the time, but I knew we should pursue it. It seemed too easy, and it was.

"Julie, has your mom taken any drugs for memory?" Eric asked when he called the following Monday.

"Yes, for just a few months," I responded.

"I'm really sorry to have to tell you this," he said, "but you're too late. We can't write it since she already has something going on."

It would be two years before I would fully comprehend the damage of this mistake—of not planning ahead for my mother's care.

Care Concept #3: Long-Term-Care Insurance and Not Keeping Problems a Secret

There will be a cure for Alzheimer's. No one is sure when. But the massive number of baby boomers about to be struck by it will drive increased governmental investment in research. Until then, step back, and thoughtfully study the options. My mother knew at some point that something was wrong. But she hid it until it was too late. We started in crisis mode instead of easing into it. Things might have been different if I had known sooner. As soon as problems are evident, people head for the doctor and throw themselves into searching—for now, somewhat futilely—for a cure. Make sure you have a plan for the future long before you are ready for it. The door to long-term care closes as soon as the diagnosis is made or the first pill is swallowed. As with any kind of insurance, you have to have it in advance in case you ever need it, hoping you never do.

We muddled through the fall, and by mid-November, things seemed to be calming down. The house hadn't sold, but Chris was handling that, and I was just the advisor when he needed it. I bought a subscription to the National Symphony Orchestra Pops at the Kennedy Center for Mom and me. As we drove home after the first one, laughing and talking about how we had enjoyed the show, I was able to see the beauty of our situation. My mother and best friend lived up the street from me. I could drive in two minutes and walk in ten. And we could go to the Kennedy Center together. I could walk my dog, Sasha, there after work.

I hugged Mom good-night in the lobby, let her walk up alone to let her feel independent, and made the short drive home to call her and make sure she got in okay. My phone was ringing as I unlocked the front door. It was Mom.

The news sent me reeling. The Renaissance had been sold and would be converted to condos. Everything had been so hard, and things were just now starting to improve. And now this? Another change? I was supposed to avoid change for my confused mother. What about the money? The angst was terrible. I had been counting on putting the proceeds from the sale of the house in the investment account. I would eventually learn that the price for the condo, even with no work being done to the unit, would be over $400,000. I sat on my stairs and cried. I thought of the verse in the Bible about God not testing us beyond what we could bear. "Okay, God," I said. "I'm pretty sure I'm at that line."

After lots of hand wringing and advice from Chris and others, I made the decision to buy Mom's unit. Over the coming years, it would at times make me look like a genius and at other times an idiot as the economy faltered and then later began to recover. But when it was all said and done, it was ideal. The change didn't happen overnight, though. There were months of legal and real-estate wrangling.

Thanksgiving rolled around, and we made plans for a family-and-friends trip to North Carolina's Outer Banks. We would drive down on Wednesday. On Tuesday, I could tell that TC was in trouble. As I mentioned, I'm a pet person from a pet family. Our pets were like our kids. But the weight of Mom's situation had me focused more on her than TC. I may have waited too long. Our vet looked a little disturbed as he said, "It's time." Mom and I held TC as they put him to sleep. I wanted to take him by myself to spare her, but she wanted to go, as she had done with our dogs in the past. It was awful. But as I would see many times later, Alzheimer's blurs the pain—for her, not for me.

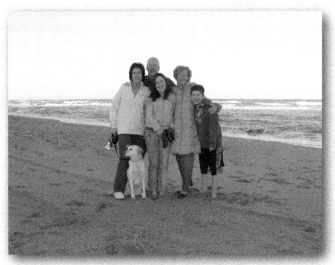

Thanksgiving at the beach

A few weeks earlier, my friend Michelle had found a cat living in the tree outside her kitchen window. The cat, who would become Charlotte, ended up with me for placement at a rescue. Charlotte might possibly be the best cat I've ever met. I knew she would get adopted quickly. That is, until we arranged for her vaccinations and she got terribly sick. "Julie, put her down," the vet had said, aware of our situation. "She's probably going to die regardless." She had a blood parasite normally found in dogs, and her future was bleak. I called Mom with the news. "We can't kill her," Mom implored. I was easily dissuaded, and Miss Charlotte, as Mom called her, spent the weekend at the emergency vet. Have you visited one before? It is more expensive than a weekend getaway for people.

On Sunday, the emergency vet called and said, "Come get her. She'll be dead if you leave her here. The only chance you have is to get her eating." Within thirty minutes of returning home, Miss Charlotte was eating and was then on major medicine for three months. After the meds were finished, Charlotte was assigned to Mom's, where she provided incredible entertainment and companionship. TC had just lain on the couch for the years he spent with Mom. Charlotte ran, chased, somersaulted, and cuddled. As I write this book, she is curled nearby. I call her the miracle cat.

>>> Care Point 3 <<<
Pets are incredible companions. Consider having one with your loved one, but plan on having an addition to your own family when the time comes.

Michelle contributed a lot more than a cat. "Jul, hold on loosely," she had said early on. It stuck with me, and I thought about it frequently. "Don't hold on so tight that you crush something special" is what it meant to me during this time. Later I found a wall hanging with something similar: "Hold on loosely; be prepared for anything, and accept that you will still be unprepared for everything." That was proving to be quite true.

During a visit from Chris and the kids, we were all laughing and talking at a restaurant while we waited to order. "Pass the rolls, please," Chris requested. Mom passed them dutifully, but as she did, she managed to feel every roll before taking one as they went by. Chris looked horrified and gave me a glance that said, "Do something!"

"I'm not allowed to touch the food I'm not taking," Rick said. I laughed. I didn't tell them that this was nothing compared to the other things I was witnessing. I had bigger battles to fight.

Don't Mess with My Mom

We waited on the condo sale. Mission One became getting Mom the best parking spot possible, since they were going to be put up for sale with the units. I wanted Mom to have the one next to the front door—close enough to be protected from the weather, but in reality, it was so my mother could find her car. I knew she couldn't keep trying to remember where she'd left it the day before, and I didn't want the management company to get suspicious. I called every morning to see if the spots were being released, and after about twenty calls, they said yes. Some other buyer had beat me to the phone that morning and bought the first two spots. But at least I had number three from the door. We got it committed to memory in time.

I saw for the first time the need to aggressively protect my mother. One of the investors tried to tell us that the terms of the contract we had signed were incorrect. I remember studying him and saying deliberately, "Don't mess with my mom," in a measured and intentionally threatening tone. Really, I was thinking, "Don't mess with me, or I'll call my brother," but my words were effective, and they backed off. I didn't know how fierce a protector I would need to become.

CHAPTER 5

Living Life

And so things went. We became owners of the condo. We settled into a routine. I was sick every time I read an article in the paper about a missing senior. The person always had dementia. Would my mom do that? And when? The idea of her being missing terrified me. I thought about how easy it would be for her to take a wrong turn and end up in Philadelphia. Or just southeast DC—not the place for a lost, elderly woman. I purchased a car tracker that allowed me to search for Mom's car on the Internet. I was watchful and vigilant in anticipating issues and studying Mom for changes that would push us into the next crisis.

It came on a sunny spring day when we both had dentist appointments. I had never stopped seeing our family dentist from my childhood, and Mom fell right back in with him. His office was in our old neighborhood—cemented, I thought, in Mom's long-term memory. I mention long-term memory again because it's so important to understand this. When Alzheimer's first attacks, it goes after the short-term memory. The long-term survives a long time. The plan was for me to see Dr. Rice first. Mom would come a little later, and I would cross paths with her as I headed to work.

I had a heavy feeling as I walked into the lobby after my appointment. No Mom. I asked Norma, our old friend and long-term employee of the dentist, if I could use her computer. Oddly, there was no Internet access on it. I bolted for my car and called one of my employees, Shannon, as I started the car. "Shannon, it's me. You have to track my mom," I shouted into the phone.

In an uncanny stroke of luck, I had just showed her the system the week before. She was able to connect quickly. "She's on Ox Road," Shannon said. I knew what Mom had done—she had exited the highway at the right place and then passed the old neighborhood. I drove around frantically with Shannon saying, "Stop. Turn around. Go back two streets. She's turned around." And then, finally, Mom and I both ended up on Braddock Road. Mom was headed east toward me, and I was headed west. "Perfect," I thought. "I'll watch for her, let her pass me, and swing around behind her." My head was swiveling as I drove, constantly looking at each passing car.

And there went her tan Camry. Just as my light turned red. "Oh crap," I heard Shannon say. "You've run through your account balance for the car tracker and I have to load more money."

"Put it on your charge card. Hang up, and call me back if she turns off Braddock."

There was too much traffic to chance running the light, so I sat, mentally figuring out how far she'd get. Green light—go very fast. I knew I was driving faster than she was and would be able to catch up if Shannon didn't call back. And then I saw them—police lights ahead on a curve. "God, please let that be Mom," I prayed. It was. I was worried about her being frantic as well as lost, and about the increasing odds of an accident. I pulled in front of her and got out. "Get back in your car," the officer yelled.

"That's my mom!" I shouted back.

He yelled, "I don't care. Get back in your car," and that time I decided I'd better listen. So I got back in my car and sat. Finally, I saw the officer approaching, laughing and looking a little sheepish.

"What did she do?" I asked. It turns out that he had seen the car tracker—a little dashboard box with an antenna—and thought it was a radar detector, an illegal product in our state. He had had his communication center quickly research it, and by the time he reached my car, he knew what it was.

I explained what had happened. He said, "Wow, you were able to track her from your car?"

"Not exactly." I explained Shannon's role. He laughed and asked if I'd been speeding. I asked if I could plead the fifth. He apologized profusely for pulling her over, and I thanked him profusely for stopping her.

The story made us laugh for years to come, and it entertained friends and many others. But the cloud got darker. My little car tracker wasn't good enough. It was hard to refresh on the Internet, and the coverage was spotty. The idea of it emptying its little piggy bank midcrisis was a problem. It was inconsistent, and I needed something foolproof until I could talk Mom into giving up her car.

The Internet yielded a better solution: a car tracker called BigBrother, which stayed active at all times and was highly reliable. Not only did BigBrother allow you to track a car, you could also set up an alert system to warn you if the car went outside a certain radius (they called it setting up an "electronic fence" around the home). The owner of the company was targeting business fleets, but I was positive he was missing a whole new market for the elderly. He agreed, and ElderTrack was born and is now available. With it installed, I was in better shape for the remaining time my mom would drive. This tracker wasn't visible, so we no longer risked the radar-detector problem. The local Toyota dealership pitched in by making the front charger "hot" all the time—meaning that the tracker would work even if the car was turned off. It just meant we would have to make sure the car didn't sit for too many days without being turned on, or the battery would run down.

Technology Tool #2: ElderTrack, by GPSAnyPlace

An ElderTrack unit is installed under the hood, sparing any confusion or embarrassment with radar detectors. It could also be installed without the knowledge of the person being protected. ElderTrack can help you locate someone who is lost or can alert you if people stray—before they become lost.

ElderTrack

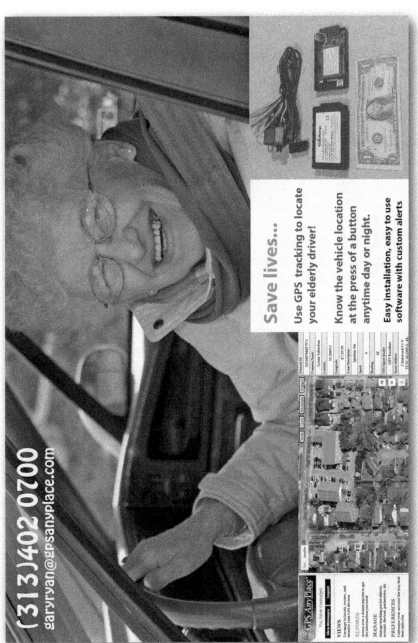

Save lives...

Use GPS tracking to locate your elderly driver!

Know the vehicle location at the press of a button anytime day or night.

Easy installation, easy to use software with custom alerts

(313) 402 0700
garyryan@gpsanyplace.com

Photo courtesy of GPSAnyplace

If at this point you are asking, "Why didn't you just stop your mother from driving?" I'm betting that you have never tried to get an elderly person to do that. Driving is freedom. Losing the ability to drive can be, I think, one of the signals that someone is nearing the end of life. I contemplated just disabling the car and letting mechanics be "stumped" as to how to fix it. But Mom was too "okay" for that, and she would have just said, "Let's buy a new car."

It wasn't long before I knew ElderTrack was worth his weight in gold. With more than a little worry, I left for my organization's annual conference in Dallas. I called Mom from the taxi for a check-in. It was six thirty in Virginia. She was always home that time of evening. But there was no answer. Miles are frightening in these situations, and I turned on my laptop. But there was her car, a little blip on my screen. She was halfway between her condo and the grocery store, headed east on Route 7 toward home. I breathed a sigh of relief as she pulled into her parking lot—all viewed on my laptop. I gave her a few minutes to get upstairs before calling. "You have good timing," she said. "I just walked in the door." I didn't let on that I knew that. She had gone for ice cream.

I never did feel completely secure. The security guards were watching at the building and ElderTrack was watching in the car, but what if she just walked away? Mom wasn't about to give up her independence in any way. There are watches that work like the LoJack system on cars, which allows the police to track a missing person. But she was wearing my grandmother's watch, and I knew she wouldn't give it up for another one. Now GPSAnyPlace offers a wearable solution as well.

When Fitness Stops Mattering

I normally went to the gym in the evening, but on the days I took off from work, I'd go in the mornings. That seems to be when older people hit the gym. They were the second wave, after the working people had begun to trickle out. The pounding beat of Survivor's "Eye of the Tiger" runs in my head every time I see them coming. *Rising up, back on the street.* They move in slow motion, which makes the song work better. *Did my time, took my chances.* They look bold and confident, and like they could eat my lunch. Which they clearly could. *Went the distance now I'm back on my feet.*

I worried about Mom's lack of exercise. Not that she'd had tons during her life, but I knew it would help her mentally and physically. But when I tried to get her to consider a fitness class, she wouldn't hear a word of it. *Don't lose your grip on the dreams of the past; you must fight just to keep them alive.* Mom was tall and thin and lucky to have had to work her entire life to make sure her weight didn't get too low. I took after my dad and have had to work to stay trim. Our doctor looked at me with a knowing smile when I told him I was worried that Mom wasn't eating enough fruits and vegetables. "Julie, why don't you just let your mom do and eat whatever she wants?" *And he's watchin' us all with the eye...of the tiger.* It was one of those early indicators that my days with Mom were numbered. I just didn't know what that number was.

Sometimes things seemed so normal. Other times, not. I developed a theory over these years: as we grow old, we become more of what we were. Cranky people get crankier, and mean people get meaner. And Mom got sweeter and lovelier. That didn't stop her, though, from smacking me one day in church. As can happen with Alzheimer's, filters get broken, and things that shouldn't be said get said. I shushed Mom in church for one of those things. And that's when she smacked me. "Don't shush me!" she said angrily. I looked around to see if anyone had noticed. I laughed to myself about how funny it really was as I rubbed the bruise on my arm, which would later have the imprint of her ring in it.

I think my summary in this book makes the whole thing sound easier than it really was. In reality, it was grueling. Every week was so short and went by so fast. I'd work long hours at work and at home, punctuated by worry, doctor visits, and crises of various sizes. The high-level pattern was to work hard during the week, knowing Mom would need me a few times; spend Saturday handling bills, finances, and other needs for two households; and then spend Sunday with Mom. I always felt guilty when people would say, upon hearing that Mom lived just up the street, "How wonderful! You must get to see your mom every day!" Well, many days. But I learned early on that I had to draw lines, or else I wasn't going to make it.

"You have to take time for yourself." How many times did I hear that from well-meaning people who had no clue? Take time? The people who said that rarely offered to help make it a reality. We all have trouble asking for help. There were times when I did ask, but it was hard for many people to take things from me and own them. But despite that, carving out time for yourself is not optional—no matter how bad things get. I looked at it this way: if I thought things were bad as they were, think about what they would be like with me not in the picture or in a hospital because of some sort of a physical breakdown.

One of the best business books I've ever read is *Getting Things Done*, by David Allen. His method of time, or personal, management helps people—especially people like me with a to-do list that could be deadly—capture and prioritize what needs to be done while acknowledging that it won't all get done. I say that his book helps you manage your schedule as opposed to having your schedule manage you. This book might not be a technology tool, but you should go buy it.

I tried hard to protect my me time. My time came in the form of dog walking and going to the gym three times a week. The dog walking was nonnegotiable, for obvious reasons. But I did a good job protecting the gym time too. There is a clear connection between mental health and physical health, and I could feel the benefits. It kept me interacting with other people, some who had been in my situation.

I Know What's Wrong with Your Dad...

One early evening at the grocery, I was pulling a cart from the rack outside when I heard a man yelling in the parking lot. An elderly man was trailing a younger man (probably my age) who appeared to be his son. "How can you do this? You can't even remember how to write a check? What do you want me to do?" He was screaming. The elderly man looked nonplussed and kept carefully walking toward the car. I was frozen. Did I run to them and try to help? Did I do nothing? I wanted so badly to say, "Wait. I know what's wrong. Don't yell at your dad." Other people stopped behind me, and we all stared quietly. I wish I could go back in time and do the right thing. Doing nothing was definitely not it. I remained frozen and they drove off, the son yelling in frustration. But for years, I kept Alzheimer's brochures in my car in case the situation repeated itself. We should always be ready to do the right thing.

Mom and I never spent much time at the condo. She always wanted to go out. For years before, she had repeated two requests if something ever incapacitated her: (1) make sure someone does my hair and (2) get me out—don't leave me someplace. And I faithfully did both. My mom was from that generation of women who got their hair done every week. On the days in between, she would glue it with hairspray. But she always pulled the technique off and looked beautiful. And out we would go—to restaurants, the Kennedy Center, drives, and fun getaways. For another of my organization's conferences, I flew Mom to San Diego with me, depositing her with Margaret and then returning at the end to spend a couple of days. But I could tell it had been hard on Margaret. I knew it would be the last visit to California.

I am pretty sure Mom knew she was in trouble and worked hard to hide it, until hiding became believing. I can't help but wonder about how different things might have been if she told me when she started to struggle. I hear from others that this is the norm. Instead, we should ask for help and start planning when it hits us. There is no time to lose.

I can't begin to count the number of times people—typically older women—would come up to me when I was with mom, put their hands on my shoulders, and say, "Enjoy these times." I would return their smiles and think, "Really? Really?" Enjoy being my mom's caregiver, protector, and guardian? I didn't *want* to do that. I wanted to be my mother's daughter and her best friend and get our old lives back. Enjoy these times? It got harder as Mom deteriorated. But now I'm thankful for these people, because they did make me pause and slow down. Their words would wake me early on April Sundays and prompt me to pack Mom up for a trip downtown to see the cherry blossoms. Or cause me to linger after lunch with her and enjoy another cup of coffee so we could talk.

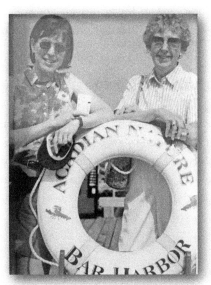

Mom and me on a wonderful trip around the northeast

The Perfect Gift

Patricia, a friend and colleague whom I greatly admire for her creativity and energy, gave me a wonderful gift around this time. "Your yard has so much potential," she said. "Let's make it beautiful." And out came a design that, when it was finished, was so beautiful it was embarrassing. I had unintentionally surpassed every other house in the neighborhood—so much so that cars would roll to a stop out in front, and neighbors would study her work. Patricia's gift was the most special one I received during this time. It was truly "the gift that keeps on giving." Each year, it would (and still does) get prettier. Even in my frenetic state, I could take ten minutes in the evening to have a glass of wine on the deck. Sasha would join me. I would stare down at the beautiful shrubs and flowers, and Sasha would watch people and wild animals.

We should be creative when we care for hurting people. Patricia was, and it changed me. During my time caring for Mom, I frequently thought back to times when I wasn't there for people who needed me. I was absorbed in work and in watching out for my mom. So why was I surprised when some friends fell away? But the ones that counted stood firm, showed up, and were creative. Michelle frequently sent cards and letters. Another friend named Ann would say, "I have two hours to do whatever you need me to do" and show up. Patricia did the garden, and our other friend Pat helped all the way along, as you'll see later in the story. John, Barbara, Ruth, and Keith kept taking Mom out for ice cream, lunch, movies, and coffee regularly for years. My parents' friendships were so strong, so invincible, that they had transferred to me.

Care Concept #4: Invest in Lifelong Friendships

Friendship investments are just as important as financial investments. Cultivate them early and often by showing up, giving creatively, and offering support. Don't let busyness lead you to sacrifice this key part of life. Your true friends will be the ones who stick around when it gets ugly—and the new ones who join you in the midst of struggle.

CHAPTER 6

Warning Signs

did something that turned out to be brilliant. I am not brilliant, but it was truly a great idea. Mom was a voracious reader of all different types of books. But like me, she would read them only once. So her book piles grew. And she was passionate about helping others. "Mom," I said one day, "why don't we bring your old books to CARE-Assist? I bet the people who live there would really like them." CARE-Assist is a national, higher-end assisted-living chain. Mom beamed. She loved the idea. So on a Sunday afternoon, we drove to one of the locations near us. Our visit was unscripted and unplanned. And it was beautiful. A woman greeted us at the door. It was homey, and a large group of residents was gathered in the nicely decorated dining area. An older woman, who I learned later was a resident, was banging out tunes on the piano, and everyone was singing along.

I was stunned. Mom stood at the doorway swaying to the music and then started clapping. Something very important was happening, I was sure. And with no prodding from me, Mom headed for the piano. I stood at the doorway on purpose and let this be her thing. They sang and sang—patriotic songs, songs from Mom's childhood. As the event began to break up for dinner, Mom came over to me and said, "Let's do this again." Bingo. And I had intentionally brought only one bag of books, leaving more in her living room. My plan was beginning to form.

When you have a problem, you tend to connect with others who have the same problem. Or who had it. At work, while dog walking, at the grocery—they popped up everywhere. A common theme was a woman named Helen Carter. "You have to learn more about her company," people would say. So I did, and I learned that there is an entire industry out there focused on seniors. They provided consulting to the elderly and to "kids" like me; they employed "companions" (people who come over several times a week to visit, go to lunch, grocery shop, or do whatever is needed); and they employed caregivers (people who did more care-related functions for people like my mom).

"I Don't Need You to Find Friends for Me"

I met with a small team of CARE-Home employees (including the owner herself) early one morning. I could tell they had been doing their jobs for a long time. The offices were frumpy and the technology outdated, but they had a lot of experience, and based on the recommendations, I decided to work with them. Our first CARE-Home employee was Cindy, an American-born woman whom I came to adore. I mention "American-born" here because in Washington, DC, most caregivers, and thus most of the employees of CARE-Home, were from western Africa, particularly Ghana.

Mom hated Cindy at first. "Julie, I don't need you to find friends for me," she would say. I lied and told her Cindy was a friend of Pat's and needed a job. Grudgingly, Mom would go places with Cindy. Cindy was a pro, and after several months, they settled into a routine. Eventually Cindy got to know me well enough that she would make decisions on my behalf—at the doctor, on clothing, with Mom's credit card.

One night after work, Sasha and I walked to Mom's, and we sat in the living room talking. My dad always said that my mom and I could talk about nothing for three hours and then repeat ourselves. I had inherited her gift of the gab, and it was fun. I noticed something on her balcony and went out to see what it was. It was a warped and melted microwave container—the kind that frozen lasagna comes in. Mom had clearly put it in the oven. I had resorted to buying her microwave dinners for use when she wasn't with me, since using the oven was a little tricky. Mom didn't like to cook anyway. She'd enjoyed it when she was raising her family, but when I hit college, she hung a sign in her kitchen that said "Let's eat out."

"Hey, Mom, remember that you only need to use the microwave." I had instructions for the microwave taped to the door. In hindsight, I should have unplugged the oven.

"I think I've been on this earth a little while longer than you have, and I don't need you to tell me how to cook," was her response.

I was learning to not react to these little quips. "I'm just worried you could start a fire if you put a microwave container in the oven."

Mom looked at the twisted piece of plastic in my hand and said, "I did not do that."

I had to hide my smile. My mother was lying to me. And it wasn't a good lie. Like someone else was going to drop a melted container on her sixth-floor balcony? "Well, I didn't do it," I said. Mom laughed. She was busted.

There were a few similar incidents, and my radar was up. I couldn't let Mom put others or herself in danger. A few weeks later, Mom called me to tell me the toilet was stopped up. I headed over with a plunger in hand, but something didn't look right when I got there. As in, what was in the toilet wasn't what one would expect. I never knew for sure, but it looked like a combination of coffee grounds and kitty litter. Again, I had the sixth floor in mind. Five units below us that we could flood if something went wrong. "Mom, would you promise me you won't put anything in the toilet?" I asked.

Mom looked at me and with a familiar refrain said flatly, "I didn't do that."

"Well, don't look at me," I said. Mom laughed, and once again she knew she'd been caught.

Criminals—Illegal and Otherwise

I became increasingly aware of the criminals and "barely legitimate" people who were out to get my mother and other seniors. It was the "barely legitimate" ones who caused me the most concern. Mom and Dad were very giving people and had raised me to be generous with my money and my time. I didn't worry at first when I saw that Mom was giving small amounts of money to some no-name nonprofits. Then I started answering the phone at her house and realized how frequently they were calling her. One day I pretended to be her and was horrified at how the caller pretended to be her friend, hoping she would continue supporting his organization. They were mailing too—about five organizations—and they were thanking her for her contributions. I was done. I studied the documents they had mailed, and in the very fine print, I read that the gifts were not tax deductible. "Fundraisers," I fumed. It was clear someone was pocketing the money.

With coffee in hand one afternoon, I picked up the first notice and dialed the number. I was firm. "I want my mother off your call list and off your mailing list, got it?" I had already put her on the Do Not Call Registry, but that seemed to have questionable results.

The man on the other end of the line said, "Will do."

I picked up the second notice and dialed the number. Different number, but the same man answered. "Oh, I believe we just spoke," I said.

"Look, lady," he said crossly, "I have five organizations, and I'll take your mother off all five of them."

Suddenly I could see his game. "Do you target the elderly?" I asked calmly.

"Lady," he said, "I can't help it if it's the elderly who like to support my causes."

"How do you sleep at night?" I asked, still calm.

"I gotta make a living," was his response. "I'll take your mother off all my lists. Have a nice day."

"Have a nice day?" I fumed as I hung up. "Have a nice day?" Researching the company online, I found that it was selling franchises around the country—franchises to seek donations, keeping ninety cents of every dollar donated. They were probably legal, I surmised, but in my mind they were unethical.

The following week, the CARE-Home nurse came for a planned visit. I went to work late so I could be there, knowing that she was going to give my mom what is called a "mini mental." Mom had been given a number of these tests by her doctor—a list of basic questions that normal people know. Mom had been steadily dropping in her ability to take them, and I had an ominous feeling about this one. I told the nurse and Mom that I would be in the kitchen. Not wanting to make Mom nervous, I clanged pans and glasses together to sound like I was busy. And I listened.

Get the Car and Get It Now!

"Who is the president?"

"What year is it?"

"What is your daughter's name?"

Mom was failing question after question. I leaned on the counter with my head in my hands and knew without any word from the nurse that we had turned a corner. As we walked out together, she said firmly, "Get the car and get it now. Your mom is acting like she knows what she's doing, but she's too confused. What if she backs over a mother and a baby stroller?" How dumb was I that I hadn't thought about this aspect sooner? The liability in addition to the heartache? I had clearly waited too long and had to move fast.

> >>> **Care Point 4** <<<
> Remember that letting an incapable person drive isn't only about him or her—it's also about the people he or she might injure. And it could be about lawsuits.

Enter our ophthalmologist. Coincidentally, we already had appointments. I called ahead and talked to him about our situation. I asked, "No matter how good Mom's vision is, will you fail her? You don't actually have to do anything—just say that you'll need to report her to the state." Mom was terribly afraid of driving tests after having to take them regularly in California. I'm not a fan of intrusive government, but I do think that the California policy is a great idea. The test threat would scare Mom.

It worked. "Betty," the doctor said, "I'm afraid you didn't pass your eye exam. I'm going to need to report this."

For over a year after that, Mom would say that she was contemplating taking the driving test and proving she could drive, but I knew she never would. She would tell people it was her decision to just stop driving instead of taking the test. The timing was perfect. Erica was turning sixteen, and Chris and I bought the car from Mom and gave it to Erica. She would love that car as much as Mom did. And it was out of Mom's sight.

Things were changing, and I needed to know the next steps. I learned early on that I felt better having facts—and having them before I needed them. Back came my planning skills. Mom couldn't live alone any longer.

Analyzing Options

In my mind, there were just two options: keeping the condo and getting a full-time caregiver, or moving Mom to an assisted-living facility. By this time, we had made a few more trips to CARE-Assist with books, and it was feeling very homey. Plus, I knew that I would be very involved, which meant it needed to be close. The CARE-Home staff were not fans of CARE-Assist for a variety of reasons. A primary one they gave was that it was very corporate.

"What's the negative?" I asked.

"Well," one of them had said, "a resident fell out of an upper-floor window at one of the locations."

I was horrified and actually remembered reading about it in the paper. But with my practical, business background, I said, "Yeah, but I bet it only happened once!" The idea of corporate rules, policies, and procedures just didn't sound like a problem to me. I didn't know then exactly how right I would turn out to be. So I was comparing CARE-Assist to in-home care provided by CARE-Home. I now knew them, and they knew me. Why would I get help from anywhere else?

It was a basic analysis, and it looked like this:

	CARE-Assist	CARE-Home
Monthly Fee	XXX	
Caregiving		XXX
House Payment		XXX
Insurance		XXX
Condo Fee		XXX
Utilities (electricity, phone, cable, water)		XXX
Food		XXX
Necessary Repairs		XXX
Incidentals	-same-	-same-
Total	$XXX	$XXX

I'm not filling in the exact numbers because they vary so widely around the country, but you get the picture. In a facility, the costs are rolled up into a monthly fee. At home, we would face additional expenses, with some being unknown (like unplanned repairs).

The decision based on this analysis was pretty easy at the time—CARE-Assist was cheaper. In-home care was the most expensive by a fairly significant margin. However, I'll jump ahead here and say that this comparison changes as someone needs more help. Assisted-living facilities typically have a basic fee for someone who doesn't need much oversight. The more oversight required, the more the cost increases. After two years, our table had almost flipped.

Count on annual cost increases with whatever route you take. And let me say here, if you and your loved one don't have the kind of funds to do either of these options, read on. The tools we'll discuss later still apply to everyone, regardless of income. Although income may limit your options, be sure and identify all of the ones that exist. There were more than I realized at the time.

Other people would have more options than I did—moving in with kids, in-home care by family members, and so on. I was more limited because I was single and had to work. But I did miss one option. If I had considered it, my level of worry would have been lower. The option I missed went back to that night Mom called to tell me the apartment building was going condo. We would learn later that investors would keep some units as rentals. What if we had just rented her apartment back, or even moved to another apartment building? The savings would have remained invested in something other than real estate. My decision making would not have been based on the nearly half-a-million-dollar condo we were dragging along behind us. And thanks to the economy, its value would drop dangerously—I hoped for the short term.

Care Concept #5: Know Your Care Options

Be creative in looking at your options before you get to the cost-analysis stage. You probably have more than you think. Your list should include the following:

- Moving in with you
- In-home care (agency-provided caregiving)
- In-home care (private caregiver employed by you)
- In-home care at a rented apartment near you (agency-provided or private)
- Combination in-home care and day care
- Combination moving in with you and day care
- Shared in-home care
- Assisted-living facility

If you choose a facility, look for the kind with "step up" care, with a level of care that changes as the needs change. Otherwise, you will continue to move. If you choose in-home and obtain a caregiver privately, consider having a

CPA firm handle payroll to make sure your legal obligations are met—don't let this issue cause additional problems. Research each option fully.

On numerous occasions during this time, people asked questions like, "Well, how much of your mom's care do you have to pay for, and how much does Medicare cover?" How I longed for the days when I thought that the government might be a resource. It is not. Medicare does not cover caregiving. If you are looking for government assistance, you have to run out of money and then let Medicaid take over. But that can be pretty dicey. The quality is a question mark at best. And I just had one parent to worry about at this point, not two, where one parent could run through savings and leave the other with nothing.

Money is a complicated thing. I hear story after story about serious arguments between siblings over how to handle it for their parents. This is a key point for us all as we plan our financial futures: make our wishes clear, and use trusts and other legal avenues to make sure what we want to have happen is what actually happens. The money was my mother's money, every penny of it. Early on, I would have fleeting thoughts about how Mom and Dad had wanted Chris and me to have a good inheritance and to use it for our own security in retirement. Subconsciously, I had looked at it as additional security for me as the unmarried daughter with no kids. We need to fight that tendency and let our parents use all of their money if necessary, looking only at what is left over when it is truly left over. My other challenge was balancing the tendency to want to skimp and save Mom's money out of fear of running out. I wanted her to be happy. So I looked for balance on a monthly basis. But I worried every day.

By the time we reached this point, the economy had crashed, and even in the protected world of Washington, DC, home values had dropped. Condos were hit particularly hard. The value of the condo was virtually cut in half, and my worry was at an all-time high. But between our savings and what was left of the condo's value, we were attractive enough as clients to CARE-Assist.

Walking Sasha one evening, I ran into a neighbor—a single mom with a teenage daughter who was renting a house on my street. The conversation turned to parents, and I told her about my plight. She told me how unhappy she was with the house she was renting. "Would you rent the condo to me?" she asked.

"Would I? Of course!" We agreed on a two-year lease, with her paying a little below market because (a) I knew she was a good tenant, and (b) the two-year lease meant I wouldn't soon have an empty condo that was hemorrhaging precious dollars while I sought a new tenant and tried to hold everything together.

Now I had another major obstacle: that independent woman I adored. How would I convince her to move in with a bunch of old people?

CHAPTER 7

The Next Move

R emember, I did something brilliant accidentally. Those book deliveries were paying dividends. Mom told my aunt Gloria (one of the cousins with whom she'd been raised like a sister) how she was enjoying the visits. And I devised my plan. Gloria would call Mom and tell her she had just seen a story on CARE-Assist on the news. "There was a long waiting list, and people needed to sign up early if they had any hope of getting in." This time, I paid CARE-Assist a visit alone. I looked at the various floor plans (knowing I already had my cost analysis) and what was available. Once again, the perfect unit was waiting. Empty.

Gloria made the call. Mom called me to tell me I'd better put her name on the fictitious waiting list. I called Chris and told him to get ready to move again. Fast. CARE-Assist couldn't give me long, but they promised not to let the unit go without calling me. I made one more trip to CARE-Assist with Mom under the guise of making sure they were looking for the unit she wanted. She agreed, but more because she was trusting my judgment a lot by this point. She knew she couldn't remember things.

As we stood in the unit and were given an overview by an employee, Mom looked at the tiny oven. "Does it work?" she asked.

"No, they are all disconnected for liability purposes," was the response.

Mom said she'd never move someplace without an oven. Knowing Mom would always vote for the dining room, I said, "I'll pay the fee and make sure it's connected."

"You'd have to sign major paperwork taking responsibility for a fire," the employee whispered as we left.

"Don't worry," I responded quietly, "We won't turn it on, and she'll never know. She won't be opening the oven door." I knew for sure about this.

In a repeat of the Renaissance call, we waited a week. "Make the call," I said to the manager, who was very supportive of our effort. Once again, Mom said *no*. Once again, I said, "It might not come again." And once again, Mom gave in. We had another downsizing to make and another moving strategy to accomplish.

The Less Stress, the Better

Mom was still Mom at this time. Although her short-term memory was pretty bad (and her long-term memory was showing warning signs), she was still herself. She knew what she believed and how she felt about things. It's just that the discussion would drop out of her memory. Thus, repetition became the big problem. We took it in stride. Sometimes Chris would make me laugh because he would say things like, "Mom, it's like I was just telling you…" I, on the other hand, would just explain things repetitively.

We had learned well that the lesser the stress on Mom, the better. So the night before the move, I brought her to my house for the night. Chris and I met at the condo and packed like crazy. This time, I knew exactly what would fit. I had measured the furniture and put blue painters tape on the floor at CARE-Assist. Why had we moved ten pillows and fourteen blankets from San Diego? I chuckled at what I'd learned over the last few years.

Pat picked Mom up early the next morning, turning her over to Ruth and Keith in the afternoon. And so started the next transformation, again making sure that pictures fit and the furniture looked as normal as possible. My friend Lisa was stationed at my house, someone else was stationed at the condo, and I was stationed at CARE-Assist. A moving company shuffled between the three stops (four including Chris's truck). By now, we were down to very special items.

I learned something during our multiple downsizings. That is that we need to distinguish between "special" and "meaningful." Every picture, every flowerpot, and every trinket was special. After all, my grandmother had touched and loved many of these things. But one could feed hoarding tendencies if left unchecked. I knew that it wouldn't be long before all the remaining items ended up at my house or Chris's, and I didn't want to have a sad shrine to my family. So I tried to think of what really mattered—and what mattered to Mom.

>>> **Care Point 5** <<<

Learn to determine between special and meaningful. Don't lose yourself by filling your home with what used to be.

We made a big deal about the introduction when Mom came to her new home. We went for dinner that night to keep it normal, and the only difference was that I slept on an air mattress in Mom's little living room. The next morning, we got ready and went down for breakfast. Mom was nervous, and so was I. I felt like a mom sending her kid off to kindergarten. People stared at the new addition who had her daughter in tow. At my request, CARE-Assist had done a little rearranging to put Mom at a table with people like her, and it helped. We all started to talk and learn about each other.

No One Is Safe

I wouldn't trade anything for the people I met at CARE-Assist. They had a knack for making you forget your troubles. Life slowed down, and worlds became small. One man took to calling me Peaches because of my fair complexion (frequently described as peaches and cream). I loved it. One morning I strolled out of Mom's unit to ask a nurse a question, and a lovely woman who was dressed to the nines stopped me. "Pardon me, darling, but could you tell me where the dining room is?" She was clearly one of the building's upper-class residents. I guess Mom was upper middle. I smiled and directed her to the stairs and the right direction. As I headed back to Mom's ten minutes later, there she was again. "Pardon me, darling, but could you tell me where the dining room is?" Uh-oh. Dementia clearly does not discriminate based on income level. Off again the perfectly coiffed woman went. She reminds me today of the randomness of the disease. No one is safe.

The next few days were a little bumpy, but overall, things went well. Mom learned to find her unit. We arranged for a locking door to protect her belongings, and we must have gone through ten keys during the time she was there. She wore a band on her ankle (where no one would see it), which would lock the exit doors and trigger an alarm if Mom got too close—another mini mental had determined that CARE-Assist wasn't comfortable with her mental state without it. I was supportive. Although it probably wasn't foolproof, it was a big safety improvement.

One day, CARE-Assist called to tell me Mom had cut her ankle bracelet off. Although I had told her everyone wore one so they could make sure everyone was safe, Mom still hated it. I drove over. Sure enough, Mom was braceletless.

"Hey, Mom," I said, "you have to keep that bracelet on or else I get a call."

"I didn't take it off," Mom said.

I had to laugh. "Well, how did it end up here in the wastebasket then?" I asked, taking it out and holding it up.

"I did *not* put it there," she reiterated. I knew Mom had been out with John and Barbara that day, so I gave them a call to see if they knew how Mom had ended up with scissors. (I had confiscated all of them when we moved.)

"Oh no!" Barbara exclaimed. "Your mother told us she wanted to buy some scissors for you as a gift, so we stopped at the store on the way home." Gee, she was getting good at this lying thing. Barbara and I still laugh about this.

Charlotte was welcome at CARE-Assist, but the risks worried both Mom and me. Management offered to put a bracelet on her to prevent her from getting too close to a door, just like Mom. But the likelihood of her slipping out of Mom's unit and through an exterior door worried both of us too much. So Miss Charlotte moved in with me, and we all settled into a new routine.

CHAPTER 8

Chasing Criminals

tell people now that there were two crimes at CARE-Assist, but there were really three. Within weeks, my grandmother's ring, which had always graced my mom's right hand, was gone. I knew she hadn't lost it—she still remembered things like this, and her daily routines were solid. I searched every nook and cranny of the unit to be safe, but my heart sank. It was gone. CARE-Assist had repeatedly stressed that we should not keep valuables there. But how do you take what is special from your mother? This is a key thing to think about when you make this decision. I never thought to take a picture of it so that the police could have searched local pawnshops. But that was one step I regrettably skipped. Nothing would come of it, and I had to move on. That was the first crime.

>>> Care Point 6 <<<
Limit valuables that get sent to assisted living. To protect what does go, take pictures in case of theft. But remember that the thief could also be a wandering resident.

Mom and I worked out a routine to manage her cash. Every Sunday evening, I would make sure that she had forty dollars in her purse. Her friends normally put expenses on her credit card when they took her out, so she didn't need much. But having cash was important to her. It took a while to settle into this routine, but it finally happened. And then, within weeks, Mom started calling me in anger, telling me that I had not given her enough money.

"I think someone might be stealing money from Mom's purse," I told Chris one evening.

"Watch it," he advised. "I'll handle it if you're right." A police detective, he was all cop. But when his mother was involved, look out. My brother was aggressively protective of his family.

A couple more weeks went by, and there were a couple more indicators that something was wrong. So I started watching more closely. I knew when I was giving her the money. Before breakfast, I would call and ask her to check her wallet.

"How much money do you have?" I would ask.

"Forty dollars," Mom would say. Then I'd call back after breakfast and repeat it. Her answer was always the same. Until a few days later. Mom exploded in anger and chastised me for not giving her enough money. There was nothing in her wallet. Now I knew. Money was being stolen.

Chris came up the following weekend, and we had a family meeting to discuss what to do. In the end, it was unanimous: we would get a camera and use it to protect her for the rest of her days. But we sat quietly for a while as Mom contemplated the decision we were asking her to make. And we wanted her to make it. Much of her life would now be on video, but I would be the only one to see it—unless we caught a criminal, in which case only the relevant parts would be seen by others. Mom had been cautious all her life, and she knew that this was necessary. Chris and I agreed after she announced her decision. She didn't want people taking advantage of her or taking her things.

Chris was never one to do anything halfway. He was researching cameras, and only the best would do. When the camera made its way to me after he handled the setup, the first thing I noticed was that it came from Israel. Well, no one is better at security than Israel, right? It was a large jewelry box suitable for an elderly woman, and it had a working clock in the front. Even I couldn't see the pin-sized hole in the clock. But open the little door and there it was. To me it was obviously a camera, and we were in trouble.

"Just back off," he would say. "You know it's a camera, and you are too focused on it. No one but the three of us will know. Criminals never notice stuff like this." I knew the detective was right.

And then began the morning routine, calling before and after breakfast. We had to wait a week before Mom's answer was, "I'm out of money again!" I bolted for the door with my laptop in hand, once again running late to work. The camera had a small card, readable by a USB device plugged into my laptop. I studied the pictures carefully, and there she was. A caregiver whom I recognized, chatting with Mom and closing the door as Mom left for breakfast. Then she calmly opened the closet door, took Mom's purse from the shelf where we always kept it, and removed the cash. I gasped—I knew I would see something like this, but it was still shocking. I called Chris to tell him I had a video but that I thought it was too fuzzy. I work with attorneys enough to know that a questionable video would not convict our thief. It would have been enough for CARE-Assist to fire her, however. We decided to stay quiet and wait.

Technology Tool #3: Nanny Cams, sold by Nannycamdirect. com (and others)

> A camera or camera system is essential when you have a nonfamily caregiver in your home or the home of a loved one. Nanny cams are easy to set up and are inconspicuous, coming in the form of smoke detectors, air purifiers, clocks, radios, and numerous other everyday products. But nanny cams show only what happened. They provide no advance protection and offer no "threat benefit" simply by being visible. You will also need to be able to access the camera without being seen to remove its camera card. Many people can install nanny cams on their own, but installation assistance is also available. Nanny cams require less of an investment than full camera systems.

This effort was not just about Mom. Intuitively, we knew that our criminal was victimizing the other residents as well. They just didn't know it. And not everyone had kids as devoted as we were. Chris contacted his peers at Fairfax County and gave them a heads-up on what we were doing. They all agreed that we needed a good video, so I went back to work on my calls and money questions. A week later, it happened again. I bolted over. This time, the results were crystal clear. The light was on, and in a stroke of luck, our thief looked at the clock to see what time it was while she was holding Mom's purse, the wallet, and…the cash. It was perfect. I called Chris, and he set me up with the detectives. After a brief discussion with me, they were on their way. I was rattled. "Could you not look like police when you come?" I implored.

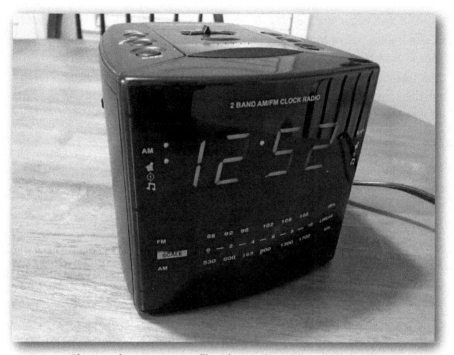

The second nanny cam—you'll read more about it later in the book.

That didn't work. Detectives Allen and Warhaftig were obviously police, to me, anyway. As we walked past the reception desk, we pretended to chat. I felt so obvious. But as Chris had promised, no one noticed. People don't watch us the way we watch ourselves. The three of us sat with Mom in her unit and discussed the camera and the situation.

"Mrs. Nielsen, can we put some extra money in your purse to help us catch your thief?" they asked.

"Sure," was Mom's enthusiastic reply. She had always been supportive of the police, especially in light of my brother's career. Now was her opportunity to contribute, and she was all in. They put several hundred dollars of marked bills in Mom's purse so that the money would be traceable. We knew our thief had to be stealing a lot of money in the building, but she was doing so in small increments, making each theft a misdemeanor. Stealing at least $200 at a time would cross the felony line in Fairfax County.

Back to work we went. We continued with our breakfast calls, but nothing was happening. We learned later that the thief had gotten sick and missed work for a while. And then Mom started getting worried about having all that money in her purse. On three occasions, I would call, she would say the money was missing, and I'd rush over—only to find that Mom herself had moved the money for safekeeping. After three weeks, it was too hard. It was taking a toll on me, and it was worrying Mom. So Chris, the detectives, and I decided to pull the plug.

There are a number of traumatic life events in my memory. One of them is the call I made to CARE-Assist that morning. Karen, the executive director, was out of town, and I called her backup. My legs felt like Jell-O. "Hi, this is Julie Nielsen. I have some bad news…I feel terrible about this…I'm not sure quite what to say. Okay…here goes. The police are on their way over to arrest one of your employees for stealing from my mom and other residents." There. It was said.

"I'm on my way" was all the voice at the other end said.

Actions speak volumes. Within an hour my phone rang. I don't recall the person's name now, but it was a senior person from CARE-Assist. However, I do remember *exactly* what she said. "Thank you for doing exactly what you did, exactly how you did it, exactly when you did it. Thank you for protecting everyone in the building, as well as CARE-Assist." I was so relieved. I had even been thinking they might make us leave CARE-Assist. But here they were thanking me. The last thing she said as we hung up was, "We'll be there with you." And they were.

I ended up going to work instead of watching everything unfold. I didn't want everyone to know—if it wasn't obvious already—that it was my mom who was the primary victim, or that we had the camera. In a call that afternoon, Detective Warhaftig told me how great CARE-Assist was. They requested marked cars and uniformed police officers to come and arrest our thief. Later I found out that they had gathered all of the employees in one room after the arrest. "We can't tell you why one of your coworkers was just arrested," the manager said. "But let's discuss the theft policy…" I suspected that my mom was now the safest person in the building.

It turns out that our thief later acknowledged stealing from other residents—even from our friend Mary on the very morning it all went down. But she did not, the thief said emphatically to the police, take my grandmother's ring. Somehow I believed her. Why would she admit to stealing money but not the ring? Perhaps there was another thief.

Our Days in Court

Court wasn't easy. Nothing happened the first time—just general courtroom details. Then the second time our thief's attorney claimed he needed more time. One of the detectives said, "They are hoping you won't keep coming to court."

Mom was in earshot and responded, "You tell them we'll stop coming to court when hell freezes over." I'm pretty sure that the opposing attorney heard her.

Finally, our important day in court arrived. The county prosecutor quizzed me as expected. And then it was the thief's attorney's turn. One of his questions was, "Ms. Nielsen, could you have manipulated this video?"

As I thought about whether I was capable of doing this so I could give an accurate answer, the judge thundered, "Counselor, are you accusing this witness of a crime? I suggest you change your line of questioning." I stayed composed. I had testified several times before in employment cases, and I looked straight ahead and answered questions concisely. I had two videos of their client stealing from my mother, and it was clear to all that they were legitimate. Later I wondered if they'd fought the case only to ask for leniency at sentencing.

The judge was hard to read. I had done everything possible to maintain my composure. I had shown the video myself. I dreaded the idea of our thief walking away and getting a similar job elsewhere. They called us back into the courtroom, and we sat down a few rows back. (As witnesses, they had asked us to leave when other people were testifying.) Calmly the judge declared the thief guilty—there had been no jury. And then he let loose.

"Turn around and look at this family, this mother and daughter," he said. "*Turn around*," he bellowed when she didn't do it. "You have betrayed their trust, your co-workers' trust, and your employer's trust. You have made it so this family can never trust any employee at CARE-Assist again. Is *that* what you wanted?"

Her only answer was "I had another baby and didn't have enough money." Although I had a twinge of sadness for her, I thought about all of the people in assisted living who, like Mom, were on the edge. This low-paid woman thought my mother was rich, and to her, Mom was. But she had no comprehension of what would happen if that money ran out. And frankly, neither did I. I could only worry about it.

I was surprised that I had a say in the sentencing. There were negotiations between the attorney and the prosecutor and then a discussion with Detective Warhaftig and me. "They are going to agree to three hundred and sixty days per conviction, serving a month in jail for each one."

"Why not three hundred and sixty-five for each conviction?" I asked out of curiosity. The answer was that our thief's ability to stay in the country would be at risk, which would likely lead to an appeal, with the risk that the convictions could be overturned.

I knew if Chris had been at the trial, he would have said, "Go for three hundred and sixty-five per conviction, and let's get her deported." We had agreed that criminal behavior was a good reason to get escorted out of the United States. But standing there in that courtroom, I decided that going through another set of court dates would be too hard—on Mom and me both. And what if the convictions were overturned? My job, I felt, was to make sure that this woman had a record and would never set foot inside another assisted-living facility. I also wanted to scare her away from her life of crime. I turned to the detective and said, "Will sixty days scare the shit out of her?"

He answered, "Julie, one day will scare the shit out of her."

"Okay," I said.

I called Chris from the car and, as I surmised, he wasn't happy that she was not getting deported. But he had a good grasp on what I was going through, and we dropped it. Jail was good enough to send a message. Our job there was done. We would continue to joke about the camera and even wave at it. We had left the watchful eyes of the Renaissance security guards and the car's ElderTrack for the watchful electronic eye of a camera. We couldn't be everywhere. And that concluded the second crime.

⸺⧟⸺

Sue was a lot like me, and I liked her instantly. We met her and her mother (another Betty) one day when Mom and I were returning from lunch, as the two of them sat in the shade in rocking chairs. Sue's mom had more physical limitations than Mom did. We swapped stories and encouragement and quickly became friends.

After we'd been griping about something one day, I whispered without looking at her, "Mom has a camera."

"So do we," Sue whispered back. Somewhat surprised at her news, I wondered how many electronic eyes were in the building.

CHAPTER 9

Assisted Living, Part I

Despite our brush with crime, life at CARE-Assist was generally good. I knew that one bad employee did not taint the rest. And the rest were truly lovely. Management and caregivers alike were professional and well trained. That corporate approach I had banked on came through—training, practices, and policies were consistent.

On one of those early days, I respectfully pushed a manager for something Mom needed. She whirled around and said, "Look, you are not in charge anymore."

I could have been angry, but I wasn't. I stood there as she walked away, and I realized that, indeed, someone else was in charge of my mother. I wasn't in charge anymore. That could be good or bad. Much later I recounted that story to the top manager at CARE-Assist, and she was horrified at what her employee had said.

"I'm not mad," I said. "She was right, just blunt."

>>> Care Point 7 <<<
Read *Don't Sweat the Small Stuff*, by Richard Carlson. A lot of life truly is small stuff.

I was a driven businesswoman and had been the overachiever of the family. If something needed doing, I made sure it was done all the way and the result was good. But I learned an important lesson during this time, and that is you can't achieve perfection. You have to analyze the situation, make a decision, and move on. No second-guessing, no do-overs. Taking care of Mom cured me of perfectionism. That was because I just couldn't be perfect—it was physically impossible. When I stopped trying to kill myself making things perfect, the situation improved.

Here's an example. Mom was always a sharp dresser—that goes along with the hair thing. She cared a lot about how she looked "because you never knew who you might run into." In fact, she worried about me after I got Sasha and began to take morning walks with bed hair. "What if you meet Mr. Right?" she would ask.

"Well, he'd probably have bed hair too," I would respond.

But our mostly African caregivers clearly had a different taste in clothing. Sometimes when I would pick Mom up, she would emerge with some pretty unusual outfits on. In the early years, if it was really bad, I'd take her back up and say, "Let's put on something that matches just a little better." But later, I just couldn't fight that battle. And at some point, they learned to dress Mom a little more like I dressed. I must have rubbed off.

Mom was easy for everyone to love. While some individuals with Alzheimer's can become combative and downright awful, Mom was sweet and beautiful. I noticed that many CARE-Assist reports said they thought Mom was "delightfully confused" or "pleasantly disoriented." Mom was almost always happy. Someone had told me early on in this fight that Alzheimer's is harder on those left behind—they struggle as they watch people go. But the person who has it is...well...delightfully confused.

I'm not sure if it was because I was around a lot or if it was Mom's popularity, but Mom and I enjoyed a special status. Both of us were well known. I made a point of showing up at all hours of the day, just to make sure the employees were always on the ball. Parts of my schedule were very routine, but others were unpredictable.

Sometimes when I was leaving at night, there would be a small group of residents gathered over coffee and dessert. They would always insist that I join them. "Come on, Peaches," our one friend would say. "Just sit for ten minutes." It was always longer than that. I loved how life slowed down when I sat with them and we talked and laughed. I always knew I was in the right place. My favorite time to be there was for breakfast. The company was good, and so was the food. Where Mom had always been the life of any party, now she was quiet. I did the talking for both of us and helped make her part of the conversation.

Alzheimer's has such an odd, random effect. Mom was enjoying herself and getting out, and she could pretty easily fool strangers into thinking she was perfectly fine. One thing that happens to people who have it is they get their times of day reversed. Once in the middle of the night, Mom called me to ask what I was up to. "Sleeping!" I laughed. "And you really should be too."

When I recounted the story to Barbara, she confessed, "Your mom has been doing that for a while, Julie, and we just didn't want to worry you about it."

"A lot?" I asked incredulously. I wondered how many people Mom had been calling and waking. I tried to find a way to limit her phone access to waking hours, but the right way of doing that never materialized. Chris contemplated creating something with a green light for "it's okay to call" and a red light for "it's too late to call."

"I don't think Mom would remember what the lights mean," I sighed. I did see a product once for a phone that had only receiving capabilities, so others must have this problem too. But Mom was still making calls to her friends, and I didn't want to take that away. I wanted only for her to call them at normal hours.

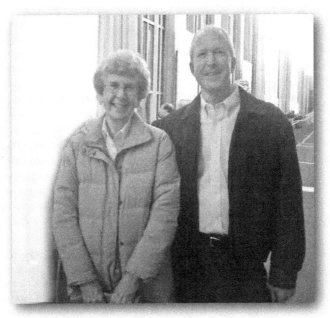

Mom and Chris share a moment at the Kennedy Center.

Making Time for Bill

MaryKate, one of the managers at CARE-Assist, caught me one day and told me about a man who had just moved in. "His name is Bill, and you really need to meet him. He used to be a pastor at your church." I agreed and said I would make a point of it. She knew my rock-solid faith, and I could tell she was intentionally connecting me with a man of similar faith.

My weeks were a blur of repetitive activity. On one particularly harried weekend, I woke up early and lay in bed thinking, "How can I get everything done today?" I contemplated skipping church and using the time. But Mom loved the church I had switched to when she moved back to Virginia. It was big and, I'm quite sure, way more modern that she would have chosen, but she loved the pastor and his preaching as much as I did. I picked the church for me, though—I had to make some decisions to benefit myself. It was where I needed to be.

"I can do this," I told myself. I decided that if I rolled out of bed fast and rushed, I could walk Sasha, down a quick breakfast, hit the grocery store and gas station, get back to put groceries away, and be at CARE-Assist to pick up Mom and run to church. Getting to church late was a big deal because of its size and the difficulty of parking, especially later when we needed easier access and handicapped parking spots. My backup plan was to bag church and go to a museum if we couldn't park.

Everything conspired against me—traffic when there shouldn't have been, lines at the grocery when there shouldn't have been, and a talkative cashier. Out I rushed and headed home. I threw cold items in the fridge and headed back out. The CARE-Assist bus was parked in front, blocking where I normally picked Mom up, so I had to park farther away.

"You're late!" she said angrily as I met her at the door.

"We need to go," I said. I had learned long before that there was no rushing my mom. In fact, when you rushed her, she moved even more slowly.

Halfway between the door and my car, trying to walk-rush Mom, I heard my name. It was MaryKate. I didn't turn around at first, thinking I wasn't up for conversation. Just get to the car. MaryKate's voice grew louder and more insistent. I turned around and said, "Hi there. We gotta go—we're late."

"I know," she said. "Bill is on the bus."

I thought for a moment, remembering who he was. "Where are they going?" I asked.

"To the Catholic church." Her words landed like a thud. We're not Catholic. I knew Bill wasn't either. MaryKate clearly understood that too, and she stared at me. I think she knew I would cave.

"Why don't you ask him to get off the bus?" I said.

Down came a nicely dressed elderly man in suit and tie, looking dapper and charming. "Hi, Bill. My name is Julie, and MaryKate told me you used to be a pastor at my church. My mom and I are headed there now. Would you like to join us?"

Bill's face brightened, and he was already headed for the car. He moved much faster than the Julie-Mom combination, and he had both of our doors open for us when we caught up. He was a gentleman. And then, as we drove the short distance to the church, he told me eight times that he was on the committee that had chosen our highly regarded pastor. I could tell Bill was just like Mom. It was another one of those times that felt right. If I'd been on time, or a little earlier, or a little later, our paths wouldn't have crossed. And as we drove under the church's parking deck, there was one empty spot waiting for us. In we went for a service that was memorable not for what was preached that day, but for the company I was with.

With my to-do list weighing heavily on my mind, I invited Bill to join us for lunch—lunch out was our postchurch tradition. This day it was Panera. He gladly accepted, and off we went.

I had left Mom and Bill at a table while I went and ordered, and as I was coming back, I heard Bill ask, "Did I tell you I fought at the Battle of the Bulge?"

"No," Mom exclaimed.

"I got frostbite and had part of my toe amputated."

"Fascinating," Mom said.

We started to eat, and Bill said, "Did I tell you I fought at the Battle of the Bulge?"

"No," Mom exclaimed again.

"I got frostbite and had part of my toe amputated."

"Fascinating," Mom said again. Uh-oh. Now I was with two repetitive people, and they were stuck in the same conversation. I think I heard about the Battle of the Bulge at least fifteen times that day, and I couldn't help laughing at Mom's identical responses. He kept forgetting he'd said it, and she kept forgetting she'd heard it.

It was a beautiful déjà vu. I sat between the two, enjoying coffee and listening as the repeating conversation continued. Periodically, Bill would insert a reference to finding my pastor. The world went on around us, and somehow the to-do list was fading. This would happen a lot—I'd be in a "to-do list crisis," and then things would happen to prevent me from getting to it. I learned to handle the real crises and trust that another day would always show up to handle the undone items.

"Would you two like to go to the nursery and help me pick out a bush for my front yard?" I asked them. Both enthusiastically said yes. So we returned to the car and ended up walking the aisles of our local nursery. Back to my house with a bush we went, and Bill insisted on helping me dig the hole. He was better at getting the shovel down deep because he was much bigger than I. Satisfied that we had experienced a full day, we headed home—to their home.

Bill would join us for church frequently. Sometimes he'd have left already, off with another church member. One day, again running late, I saw that Bill hadn't been signed out. I walked around to his room and knocked. He was dressed but was missing his trademark tie.

"Would you like to join us for church, Bill?" I asked.

"Oh sure, but I can't leave without a tie." He opened his closet, revealing a large rack of what looked like dozens of clip-on ties. I didn't know they made that many clip-ons. Bill had forgotten how to tie a tie, I knew, and someone had bought him a large supply of the easy-to-use version. I don't know why it struck me as funny, but it did. His secret was safe with me.

Mom Goes Missing

It was midafternoon on a workday when the CARE-Assist number appeared on my cell phone's caller ID. Seeing that number was always cause for alarm. I grabbed my cell and said, "Hello?"

It was Karen. "Is your mom with you?"

"No!" I was on my feet. "I'm at work. What's going on?"

"Don't panic. We think she is probably with one of her friends, who forgot to sign her out."

Don't panic? How do I *not* panic when my mother is missing? "I'm on my way. Call me if anything changes," I said frantically as I threw my things together and ran for the door.

"I'm calling the police," she said as she hung up.

I wasn't in full panic mode as I drove. It was Monday, and the odds were that Karen was right. Ruth normally picked Mom up for lunch and a movie on Mondays. But the uncertainty was unnerving. Remember, I said that this was my worst fear. But it's hard to get out of CARE-Assist with an ankle bracelet on. Someone was probably with Mom and had entered a code to exit without the alarm going off. As I pulled into the CARE-Assist parking lot, my phone rang again.

"Found her!" Karen said. She had rushed to the nearby mall theaters. "There were only two movies your mom would have liked, and the manager let me run into both. I found them in the second one."

"Did you talk to Ruth?" I asked.

"No, they were enjoying the movie, so I just walked out."

I liked Karen. She was the matter-of-fact wife of a law-enforcement officer, and the one who had insisted that our thief be marched out in front of everyone. I called Ruth that night to let her know what had happened, and we laughed at the episode. No one ever forgot to sign her out again.

Assisted Prison

Many people in assisted living are fragile. So when a bad virus or bug goes around, they go on lockdown as though it's a prison. People are confined to their rooms, and the boredom is awful. It happened once for the flu and once for some bad virus. Mom never got it, and I felt like the seclusion was almost worse than getting sick. One time, Mom had to be on lockdown by herself. She'd had a rash on her face for a couple of days. I didn't pay much attention to it until Cindy called to say she thought it was worse. After a visit to the dermatologist, we found out it was shingles. It wasn't bad. I was annoyed at the personal lockdown. "The nurse missed it, and we find it days later. And now you want to leave her in her room?" I pushed to keep her quarantine short.

During one of the lockdowns one evening, I was talking to Mom on the phone. She was frustrated because it was dark. "Why is it dark?" I asked. Mom didn't know. Before leaving that morning, I had asked them to fix a fuse that was affecting multiple lights. Clearly they hadn't. Back over I went. Not surprisingly, I found Mom sitting in the dark.

"Do you know my mom has been sitting in the dark?" I asked.

"No, but it couldn't have been long because we are checking periodically."

It was seven o'clock and winter, and the day had been cloudy. I knew it wasn't true. My mom had been in the dark a long time, and they hadn't noticed. I waited while they called for emergency service, and then I watched as the gentleman fiddled with the circuit box. I think assisted living is good most of the time, but you need to stay on your toes. I couldn't check the camera because it was connected to the same circuit. All seemed well when I left.

Rethinking Medical Tests

Without thinking about it, I scheduled a procedure for Mom when a doctor recommended it. It was one she'd been getting for a while that required specific preparation. Even with her at my house the night before, things went wrong preparing for it. It was one of my darker days. Mom was oblivious to what had happened. That night, I called Michelle from the darkness of my kitchen. Leaning on the counter, my head in my hands, I whispered in tears into the phone, "I can't let Mom hear me cry...she wouldn't understand." Of all the times I would call Michelle for support, this may have been one of the worst. We know each other so well, and she is the only person I know whose life is as crazy a place as mine. But she already had two daughters by then, was two and a half hours away, and could only cry with me and offer words of support. But Michelle's words of support were typically prayer after we hung up. It mattered.

"I'm walking Sasha," I called from the hallway so Mom wouldn't see my tears, and I slipped out into the winter night without a coat. I needed a jolt to recover. The first half of the walk, my emotions must have kept me warm. The cold felt good on my face. I must have recovered because then it was, as Mom would have said, "dern cold." My teeth were chattering when I returned, but there was now an excuse for my face to be red. I had recovered enough to keep pretending that everything was fine.

>>> Care Point 8 <<<
Think about whether medical tests, especially traumatic ones, are truly necessary.

I mention this story for one reason: it never really dawned on me to think about when to stop routine tests. Later, someone would say to me that something else would kill my mother long before cancer would. The doctor had said, "It's time for the test," and I had said okay. No thought given to it. Although what happened was worse for me than for Mom, I probably shouldn't have put her through it. I knew my mom was dying. I just didn't know at what speed.

CHAPTER 10

The Biggest Blow

I t never entered my brain that things could get worse. It was bad enough that I'd lost my dad at twenty-seven. That rocked my world. Then having my mom get Alzheimer's when I was in my early forties was shattering. So I was stunned when Chris called one night and said, "Are you sitting down?" He had had a heart attack. Not right then; it had most likely happened months before when he had a procedure on his back and while he was recovering from anesthesia. Oddly, I was probably talking to him on the phone when he was having it. I recalled vividly how he had been in terrible pain, saying his shoulder hurt, and nowhere near where he had the surgery. My brother was tough. And the tough guy was clearly in pain. His marriage had dissolved by that time, and he was dating a woman, Kim, whom I could talk to easily. Kim had been there trying to massage the pain out of his shoulder.

He recovered from the surgery but later decided to get one of those whole-body scans that are advertised in the paper. "Uh, you need to go see a cardiologist," the doctor said. "And quickly."

Based on my dad's history of heart disease, you might think we were both a little dim not to anticipate this. Chris and I were the children of a dead man, thanks to heart issues. But we always talked about how we were different—we knew more, ate better, and never smoked. Our only risk was heredity. We were clean-living kids who never touched drugs and weren't big drinkers.

Both of our lives were changed. I was already a fairly healthy eater and gym member. Now I became a very healthy eater and gym rat. But it was different for Chris—he was the one who'd had the heart attack, not me. I just had the risk, and he had the real deal. He was convinced that he was a short-timer, even though the doctors had said, "You'll probably be like your dad—you won't live to be really old, but you will live a good life." We rolled forward, me now with an eye on my brother and my mom.

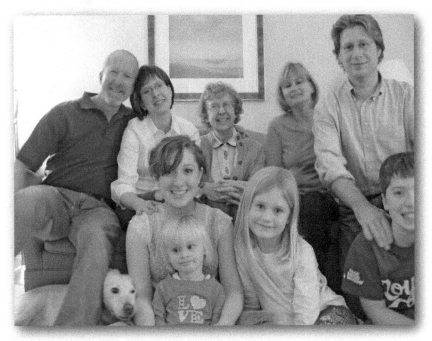

Thanksgiving 2007, the Nielsens and our close friends the O'Neills

In my world where phone calls were frequently bad news, I got a sweet one from Chris one night. He had bought a BMW. "*What?*" I exclaimed. "You don't have the money for that!" I was the bookish, practical kid who saved and planned and exercised caution. He was the kid who bought the newest and best thing, whether or not he had the money. I know he was a lot more fun as a result.

"Today could be the last day of my life, so I've decided we should live as though it is our last day," he said. "And don't worry, it's used." He loved it. Much later, when I saw it for the first time, I knew why. It was beautiful—and big. "But that's not why I was calling," he said. "I picked one out for you. I bought big and used for me. I picked a small but new one for you, and you need to come down to look at it. It's yellow."

I laughed. But the sweet thing was that he meant it—he was persistent and wouldn't drop it. I protested, "But I love my little CR-V!"

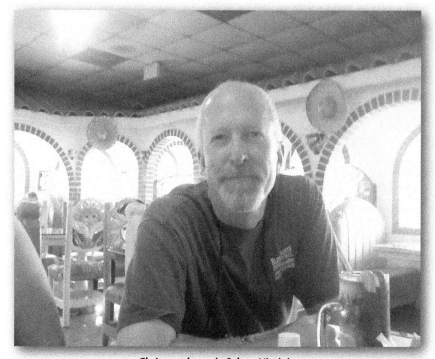

Chris near home in Salem, Virginia

It wouldn't be long before I would really understand how proud Chris was of me. "You are my successful sister up in DC. You need something nicer than a CR-V." He couldn't convince me, but I loved the fact that he tried.

I mourn, and still mourn today, the loss of the second-greatest man I ever knew. It was July 2, and I had the next day off before the holiday on the fourth. I was still at work and beginning to think about the plan I had in mind for the next four days. I would simply get things done—I always felt better when I could do that. And then the phone rang. It was Kim. I answered with an uneasy feeling because it was an odd time for her to be calling. Her words still sneak into my mind when I let them. She was distraught, but her words were clear.

"I don't know any other way to tell you this, Julie, but your brother is dead," she wept.

Words cannot describe how I felt. "Oh God, no!" I screamed, stumbling down the hallway. "No, no, no!"

Kim had gone on, "Erica called me after he missed picking Rick up for his guitar lesson, and she couldn't get ahold of him. I went to the house and found him. I have to tell the kids."

"No," I shouted, "I have to get to Maureen; she needs to tell the kids." Maureen was the kids' mom. In a way it was a blur, but then oddly, I also remember every painful detail.

And so went the next terrible phase of our lives. Friends at work got my car and me home. I did my best to pull myself together to go to CARE-Assist and tell my mom the worst news a mother can hear—that her child is dead. Karen was waiting for us as my friend Jennifer and I pulled up.

"You don't have to tell her," she said. "You could handle it another way." But Mom's mental shape was too good. She would notice that her son wasn't calling her to check in. She would be worrying about where he was.

"I have to tell her," I said.

When life gets as hard as mine got—my beautiful family dropping from my life—you have to find humor. Mom said, "But Chris did everything. What will we do?"

Despite the tragedy we were facing, a piece of me bristled. "I am the one doing everything!" I thought. But the sadness overtook me.

I never realized all that Chris had done when Dad died. And now it was my turn. Funeral planning, obituary writing, and beginning to figure out what to do with the estate. I did it numbly. The kids and Maureen were there, and we all went through the motions. But I was his protector and executor, and the only one he'd trusted to get this right. "I need to know that you'll do exactly what I want," he had said. I had thought he was being dramatic about the short-timer stuff. He wasn't. In almost every call, he would remind me about what he wanted and what to do. Even if I had known what lay ahead when I accepted the responsibility of being Chris's executor, I still would have said *yes*. I would have jumped off the roof for my brother if he had asked me to.

Jennifer spent the night, and the next day Mom and I made the sad drive to Salem.

Residents from the entire Roanoke Valley came to the two visitations by the hundreds. The stories of how my brother had touched their lives were beautiful. He was kind and gentle in dealing with victims of sexual abuse, homicides, and other types of deaths. Mom was there with me, and people were gentle and kind with her too. Officer after officer told me Chris had "told us about his sister who was a successful smart cookie up in DC." I knew Chris was proud of his kids, but I didn't realize how proud he was of me. I was stunned when I looked at the doorway and saw Ruth and Keith standing there. We were four hours from home, and they had made the trek. Moments later, it was my old friends Rob and Susie in the doorway. The devotion of these four was powerful, and their actions required no words, which was good, because all I could do was cry.

The next day, the service was moving and funny. More stories for Chris's children, Mom, and me. I laughed as I heard for the first time that my brother had fired his weapon in the line of duty. How could he not tell me? I knew he had drawn his weapon on numerous occasions, but not that he had ever fired. It turns out that a roll of carpet had tipped over during a search, and he shot it. "Which is funnier?" I thought. "That it happened or that he didn't tell me?"

People stood alongside the streets as the procession, with a law-enforcement honor guard and motorcycles, snaked to the cemetery. Some saluted as we drove slowly by. I was numb in the back of a car. The sound of twenty-one guns again cut through the air. "Taps." I forgot to tell them that Mom hated "Taps." As we sat there holding hands, I realized that Mom didn't remember who was in the casket. She stared straight ahead, glancing over and looking more worried about me than anything else. She looked confused but not devastated. I tried to breathe. As I sat there staring at the flag-draped coffin, I knew I would be living my brother's death alone. It wasn't until Jennifer came down from DC to pick Mom up and take her home that I truly felt the gravity of it all. Kim's parents had opened up their home to us, but I moved to a hotel nearby after Mom left. "Welcome to the rest of my life," I remember thinking as I sat on the bed late one night.

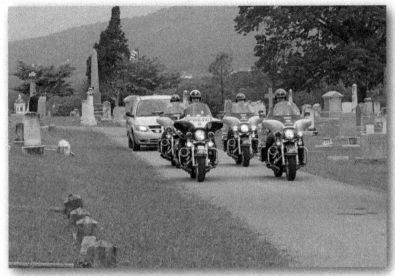

The funeral procession

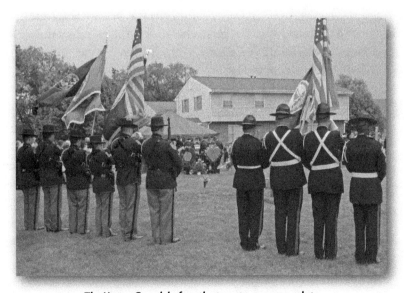

The Honor Guard, before the twenty-one-gun salute

The Margin of Life

I help other people with problems for a living. I'm a fixer. But now I was the one struggling. As was typical for me, I looked for the lesson in my life, and I found a big one. I named it the "margin of life," and I use it frequently to help others.

Care Concept #6: Manage Your Margin of Life

Maintain a healthy margin of life. If you are living at the end of your rope all the time, you will collapse if you take on more. So make changes before crises come. Because there will be crises. And if you wait, the options available to you may be fewer. If you don't address your margin of life, it could get addressed for you.

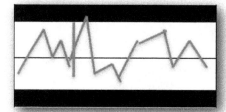

Figure 1: Healthy Margin of Life

Figure 1 indicates a healthy margin of life. A flat line at the bottom would be someone who is oddly calm and unstressed—and probably removed from reality. A flat line at the top would be someone operating at breakneck speed who is headed for a mental or physical breakdown. Note the ebb and flow around the center line. This person has room to crank up emotionally when things get tough. The vertical line indicates a crisis, and you can see the gap between the center line and the maximum.

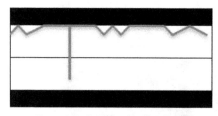

Figure 2: Unhealthy Margin of Life

Now look at figure 2. It indicates an unhealthy margin of life. This is where I was when Chris died. I was already maxed out—running on fumes, if you will. And then the bottom dropped out. There was no place to go to relieve the pressure. The vertical line in figure 2 points to the problem—it was me, pounding against the maximum. I survived, but I had to wonder what I would do on more than a few occasions.

Our challenge is to live our lives with a healthy margin of life so we can adapt in times of crisis. There will be crises. Some may find this easier to do than others. I suspect my role as a businesswoman in a major American city predisposed me to have a poor margin of life.

—∞—

Remember what I said about the difference between Chris and me? He had seven vehicles, which became part of the estate and which needed to be sold. I had no clue what to do with a big Suburban, a jeep, a motorcycle, an RV, the beautiful BMW, or assortment of trailers. Ken, an old friend of Chris's who had become a good friend of mine, helped me through with hours and hours of support and hard work. I don't know what I would have done without a strong friend to hold me up—and hold me together. Although to this day, Erica wishes I'd kept the Suburban for her.

The Big Lie

If I needed confirmation that Mom had forgotten her son's death, I got it the night I drove home a few days later, after almost a week of work at Chris's house. Ken and I had met at Chris's house that afternoon. "You need to get Salem in your rearview mirror. Your mother needs you," Ken said. Although a devastating sadness awaited me and would fill the coming months, I was optimistic as I pulled on to Highway 81 and headed north. I would be back several times to handle the estate and visit the kids, but for now, Salem was in my rearview mirror.

I drove straight to CARE-Assist to see Mom. When she saw me, her usual grin came over her face. "I'm so glad you're back!" she exclaimed. "Did you have a good time on your vacation?"

Thud. The words landed hard in my ears. I had only a second to think and hold back tears as I said the hardest words I've ever said. "I had a great time," I lied—the mother of all lies.

"I can't remember where you went on vacation," she said.

And then came another lie. "I just drove down to see Chris and the kids." It was devastating.

My friend Jennie was parked in front of my house when I pulled into the driveway. It was late, and she had a bag of groceries in her arms. "I had no idea what you'd need, so I got you what I would want," she said. We hugged through tears and unloaded the car. Not too long after, Jennie's father would take a sudden turn for the worse. He would develop a different kind of dementia and race past Mom in terms of severity. Later, when I sat in the pew in tears at his funeral, I was crying for both of us.

Care Concept #7: Stop Killing the Loved Ones

I know that sounds funny, but it's really true. People forget things when they have Alzheimer's. And they are going to keep forgetting them. So just deal with that and don't bother repeating things, especially when it's bad news. If someone died, it's as though they are dying again and again if you keep reminding the person. In my case, Chris died once. Mom forgot. I took Karen's advice—a little late—and my brother lived on. It was the defining moment of Alzheimer's for me.

CHAPTER 11

Increasing Care—and Expenses

Periodically, Mom would ask if I had heard from Chris. "Oh yeah, he said he was going to call you this weekend," I would say. The following December, we discussed what to get him for Christmas. Mom was still herself—still opinionated, and still in control of who she was. But that short-term memory…conversations and events from five minutes ago just fell away.

Shortly after I returned to work, my coworkers conspired to send me to a spa day. Without saying where we were headed, two of them drove me to a well-known Red Door location one morning, left me there, and returned for dinner. That day means so much to me still.

Not too long after Chris's death, Ken called and said, "I'm coming up. Let's figure out how to use that gun." Chris had insisted I buy a gun from him—his second-to-last service weapon, which the county had sold when it upgraded its weapons. We kept saying he would come up and spend a weekend—just the two of us—and he'd teach me how to shoot. But it never happened. And now it was going to happen with Ken.

Mom was horrified. "You're going to kill yourself," she insisted. She trusted me in all things except this.

"Chris wants me to learn, Mom," I protested, being careful to use the present tense. Ken said I wouldn't be able to shoot it—it was too heavy. "No," I insisted. It has to be this gun, the one he had carried. It didn't take long to prove I could, to Ken's surprise. And I was good. I know Chris isn't really standing next to me when I shoot it. But I feel like he is. It's as though I could reach over and touch him.

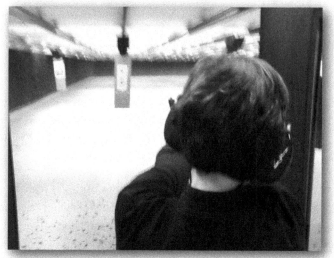

At the range with the gun Chris wanted me to learn how to shoot. So proud!

At least once a week, I would see an ambulance at the front door of CARE-Assist. I hated it. I couldn't help but know that one day it would come for my mother. Sometimes they would take people and sometimes not. And sometimes people would never come back. Despite this sad fact, it seemed to be a mostly happy place.

I was at the grocery store when the call came in. "Your mom has fallen, and we've called nine one one." I had a special fear of a broken hip, which can trigger the end for many people. I left my food in the cart and bolted for the car. "Sorry," I said as I passed a cashier. I bolted a lot in these days. I felt sick when I pulled up and saw the flashing lights. It had finally happened. They already had Mom in the ambulance, and they said to meet them at the hospital. Off we went. I could tell it wasn't bad because the ambulance was taking its time on the Beltway, with me in tow. Mom turned out to be fine, but it was the first of a number of nights we would spend at the Fairfax Hospital emergency room.

The second fall happened in Mom's room. She thought she hit the doorknob. But regardless, she hit her nose. I didn't rush this time because the nurse who called me played it down. But I was shocked when I got there and saw her. I probably would have called the ambulance that time—her nose was fat and her eyes were already bruised.

It was right before Christmas, and Mom and I were planning on going to St. Michaels in Maryland for two nights. These trips had become a tradition since Dad died. The first two years after his death, the two of us went to Hawaii—just to go someplace that wasn't traditional or too Christmas-y, since Dad had died shortly after Christmas. For years after that we would drive up the California coast to Carmel. Once Mom moved east, I picked St. Michaels as our spot—far enough to feel like you were on vacation but just an hour and a half from home.

At a local urgent-care center, I signed the forms fast—without reading them—to get Mom with the doctor as quickly as possible. As we sat in a back room, I studied a poster of the human body. "How wonderfully made we are," I thought, "when the body works and when the body doesn't work." The doctor checked Mom out, x-rayed her face, and approved our departure for St. Michaels. It wouldn't be until weeks later that I would reread what I had signed. One form said in summary, "Not only do we not take Medicare, but if you even inquire about this visit with Medicare, you agree that we can sue you." When you and your parents are healthy, you never dream that there are people and organizations like this out there. I did contact Medicare. Although they said it was impossible that a facility would do this, it was too hard to pursue. And clearly it was not "impossible." I made sure CARE-Assist and our doctor knew to avoid the place, but that was the best I could do.

>>> Care Point 9 <<<
We should always read the fine print in any document we sign, but it's especially important when it is on behalf of someone else.

Mom's nose wasn't broken, despite the swelling. So that year, she went to St. Michaels with two black eyes. I hoped people wouldn't think I was abusing her. The second day there, the bruise had run from under her eyes to down below her nose, leaving her face black and blue. But she was mostly unaware of it, and we had a good time. With all the bumps and bruises Mom suffered during this time, she never seemed to feel the pain. It was as though something had dulled.

Pretty soon, I knew there was a trend. It was early on a Sunday morning, a little after four, when I got the next call. This time I beat the ambulance. There was no traffic that time of day, and I was getting good at this. Boxer, the large CARE-Assist dog, met me at the door. It turned out that the normally silent Boxer had started barking at four o'clock. When a caregiver went to check on him, she found my mother on her back, halfway down the stairs. Thank goodness, she had fallen backward.

If you want to get out of the ER fast, go at four thirty in the morning. They were getting to know us by this time and said, "See you soon" as we left.

I am nothing if not a planner. And I'm a worrier. I don't mean I'm consumed by worry. It's just that I plan in advance for problems to happen. Sometimes they don't happen, which is nice, but I'm prepared when they do. And so it was that when Mom would come over to my house, I would make sure to leave the front door unlocked, and I would clip my cell phone on my pants. The stairs had been hard on Mom for a while. But my house felt so homey when my mother was in it. On this particular day, Pat was with us. We moved slowly, one step at a time, asking Mom frequently if she wanted to rest. Halfway up, we were in trouble. A faraway look came over Mom's face, and she began to wobble. I would see this look again. Pat had been in front, and I had been behind, but I swung myself in front of her and grabbed her. Mom landed mostly on my knee, and I held on tight and managed a controlled fall onto the stairs with Mom on top of me. Mom probably weighed about 128 pounds at this time, but that amount of weight is heavy when it's working against you—as in, someone who is trying to slide down the stairs. I was very aware of the danger of me falling down the stairs with her too. "Call nine one one," I said breathlessly as I passed my phone to Pat.

The 911 operator calmly asked Pat questions. After the third one, I took the phone and said, "Please tell me that they are on their way!"

He said, "I need to finish getting some information first."

I interrupted him rather harshly to shout, "My mother is elderly and almost unconscious, and if they don't get here fast, we could both fall down the stairs."

>>> Care Point 10 <<<
Think about what problems might happen—then try to avoid them.

In hindsight, I'm pretty sure he had already dispatched them. I hope he had. While it seemed like we were on the stairs forever, it was probably no more than minutes. Mom recovered from these episodes quickly, and they put her in my car so I could drive her home. Then they followed us so they could help get her out of the car. More great strangers. Later, when an orthopedic surgeon asked me how I tore the tendon in my elbow so badly, this was one of the possible causes I thought of as they knocked me out for surgery.

Things were getting worse. I knew it, and so did CARE-Assist.

Then Again, Maybe Not

I don't get sick much, but one spring I came down with a sinus infection and just couldn't shake it. On my second trip back to urgent care on a Saturday morning, the doctor said, "Are you under a lot of stress?"

I studied him for a moment as though he was an alien. "Well, my father and brother are dead, my mother has Alzheimer's and is dying, and I am trying to close out my brother's estate, take care of three pieces of real estate, not fall apart, and pretend at work like everything is fine. Is that what you mean?"

This time he studied me. "It's odd, isn't it," he said. "You go from loving someone to hoping every day that they die."

I was stunned at first. But I understood. I didn't want to admit it, but I constantly flipped from wanting to hold onto my mom forever and wanting her to die and get out of her worst nightmare.

"My father died from Alzheimer's a few years ago," he said. "Let's switch antibiotics. But the most important thing I can tell you is that you will make it through."

—ege—

Briefly, my friend Sue from CARE-Assist and I pondered the idea of moving our moms out and into a shared apartment. But the proposition was full of complications that we never quite overcame. I began making plans to move Mom to the third floor—the special Alzheimer's unit that was highly secure. I had visited a few times because I knew we would ultimately be headed there. It was a microcosm of CARE-Assist over-all—a beautifully decorated place with lots of things to touch and hold. The difference was that you could check in, but you couldn't check out. Security was tight. The elevators and stairways were protected. And the residents were much worse off—some wandered, some cried, some played. One woman moaned all the time. That part was awful. The sound wafted into every nook and cranny of the third floor. There was no escaping it. "I thought you said this wasn't a nursing home," I said to Karen one day.

"It's not, but the line isn't always clear," she responded. I dreaded moving Mom up there, but I knew it was time. Within days, the moaning woman was gone.

The costs were high, and I contemplated how much faster we would be running through our funds. To make matters worse, our renter had told me she was moving out and wouldn't be signing a new lease. I had plenty of notice, and I began toying with whether I should revisit the financial analysis and consider moving Mom back to the condo with a caregiver. But I liked the social activities, and so did Mom. Lunches out, movie nights. I couldn't orchestrate these things. "Don't do this to your mom," Karen had said when I mentioned the idea to her. "She needs the social stimulation." Then CARE-Assist came up with a proposal: a suite was opening up. They could modify it to make it two apartments, and then Mom and another resident they had identified, MaryJane, could share it. I'd been watching MaryJane a long time. She was somewhat ahead of Mom in her stage of the disease, and watching her helped prepare me for what I would see later. She was always laughing, which was nice. That was normally how she answered any question—with a beautiful laugh. I would laugh along.

So I agreed. But to orchestrate this move, I needed another elder fib. I was getting good at it. This time, I roped in the maintenance manager. "Mom," I began one day, "the maintenance manager told me today that a big pipe broke. They are going to have to rip out your bathroom to get to the plumbing. We're going to have to move for a few months." I knew by now that once things changed, we were set. Getting through the change would be hard, but after arrival, we would be okay.

"Oh no," Mom said, "I love my apartment. I don't want to leave it."

"They promised you can have it back," I lied, knowing we wouldn't be returning.

And on came our third downsizing. The suite was smaller still. Once again, Ruth and Pat took Mom out for the day. Ann came over, and we went to work. We did our best to make the little space look like home, but it was getting harder now. MaryJane's daughter was there too at first. "I'm afraid I have a work meeting," she said as she left, with her mother not fully moved in. The next day, I would run into her at the grocery, wearing a fresh sunburn that was hard to miss. Quite the work meeting, I was sure.

We did our best to make both halves of the suite look good. But the difference was that MaryJane was sitting there watching and worrying. It was awful. She'd laugh when we talked to her, but then she would cry and look for her things. I was fuming that her daughter wasn't there. And I had a bad feeling about the arrangement. When Mom came back that night, we went to dinner and then tried to pretend that nothing had changed, but that didn't work. I kept reminding her it was "just until the plumbing problem was fixed."

It was quiet as I was leaving, and I stood waiting for the elevator. There was commotion around the corner, and I was startled to see a naked woman bolt by me with two caregivers in pursuit. Most of the people there couldn't move that fast, but this one was agile. I hid a laugh. "Welcome to my new world," I thought. "I hope Mom never does that."

As I left, I went by the old unit. We still had items there—mostly items to discard, but I had left some breakables there for packing. I sat down on the floor to wrap them up, and that's when I noticed it. When Chris was born, Mom had bought a Hummel figurine of a boy on a ladder. When I came along, she'd purchased a girl figurine—an angel. Her plan was for them to be ours one day. I wasn't especially fond of Hummels, but they were special because of Mom's plan, and I wouldn't have traded them for anything. Long ago, the boy's ladder had been broken and glued back together. But the angel had remained safe. And now she was missing. I jumped up and tore through everything. She was nowhere to be found. I don't know when she was stolen—it could have been as the items were dwindling during the move, or it could have been earlier and I didn't notice. I was crestfallen. And furious. Although there is a chance a resident could have been our thief this time, I doubted it. Mom's door was always locked. And the thief knew to take the girl figurine and not the boy, which had clearly been fixed and would have no value. My tears this time were out of rage. It was the third crime at CARE-Assist—not as big of a crime as the others, comparatively speaking, but it hurt.

It dawned on me that the only thing of value left in Mom's possession was her wedding ring. It was a beautiful ring. For their twenty-fifth wedding anniversary, Mom and Dad had worked with a jeweler in Nags Head, North Carolina, our family beach destination, to enhance it. The engagement ring and wedding band were joined, and two other small diamonds joined the larger one in what looked a little like a crown. The idea of someone else wearing my mother's ring was too much for me to bear. I decided I would be the one to take it. Deep down, I knew my mom would agree. Back when we'd all agreed to get the camera, it was a family decision. But this was one I had to make for us.

There was a small sitting room when you first entered the suite. The bathroom was off that room as well, allowing Mom and MaryJane to be completely separate most of the time. The smell smacked me in the face as I walked in the next morning. The unmistakable smell of feces. I peeked in the bathroom, and it was all over. Backing out, I knocked on Mom's door. "We need to get out of here," she said. "It smells!" I even saw the signs of it in Mom's room. Out came MaryJane, the culprit. Her hands were covered. I was horrified. I marched Mom out the front door, holding her arms down so she couldn't touch anything. "Could things get any worse?" I asked myself. The Hummel. My increasing worry about the ring. And now this. Care managers came running when I told them, and they apologetically cleaned everything up quickly. As much as one can, I suppose. Note to self: buy lots of hand sanitizer.

The next day as I was leaving, I said, "Hey, Mom, you were going to give me your ring so I could have it fixed at the jeweler."

"Oh, that's right," she said, giving it to me.

I bit my lip to keep from crying as I headed out. I stuck it in a safe place at my house. Periodically, Mom would startle and say, "My ring!"

"Don't worry," I would respond. "It's at the jeweler being fixed." The ring was in her long-term memory, but my fictitious jeweler was in her short term.

About a week later, as things were beginning to settle somewhat, Karen caught me. "Julie, we need to put your mom in Pull-Ups."

"But Mom isn't there yet," I protested. Mom was very capable at getting around and taking care of things like this.

"The nurse said she is."

But Mom wasn't. Incontinence was one of the things that scared me. The idea of it rattled me more than any other, except maybe death. When I told Jennie of my fear one day, she had said thoughtfully, "It's not like it happens all of a sudden. There are accidents, and you work your way toward it."

I knew it wasn't true, but as I looked around, I noticed that everyone else showed the telltale bulge that indicated diapers or Pull-Ups. I got it. It was easier just to have everyone in them, and I knew that's what was happening. Not having any better options, I acquiesced. And here's where language means so much. The caregivers would say loudly to residents, "We need to put a diaper on," and residents would freak out. I would frequently intervene and say gently, "She's going to help you put your underwear on, okay?" This technique was helpful on many occasions. Choose your words carefully—nurses can be "friends," and diapers can be "underwear."

⸺◦◦◦⸺

What landed us in the ER again the next time wasn't exactly a fall. It was the underwear. I was there one day when a caregiver was helping Mom pull up her underwear in the bathroom, and Mom was resisting and frazzled—the kind of agitation that precipitated the falls. As the woman helping her tried to get her to stand on one leg on the hard bathroom floor, which in itself was clearly a problem, I saw Mom's head tilting back and that expression coming over her face. The caregiver was oblivious. "Stop!" I shouted. "She's fainting!" Mom collapsed in my arms. "Get help," I yelled, and the woman ran. It's good Mom was fairly light. I propped her on my knee and slid us both down the wall to the floor.

This time they decided to admit Mom to run tests. In hindsight, maybe we should have done that sooner, but after each of the falls, she had been fine. But this time Mom's confusion increased the hour she was admitted. This was the first time I ever heard about how people as young as fifty get, well, "wacky" when they are admitted to the hospital. I saw it right away. Mom was insisting on leaving and kept trying to get out of bed. Then she wanted to know what my wedding dress looked like. I knew we were in trouble. I was hopelessly single.

"I need help," I told the nurse. "My mom is fragile and confused, and I won't be able to keep her in bed."

"Let me see if I can get a sitter—but I doubt it."

I tried to stay alert. Mom would doze. I would doze. Then I'd wake up with a start as she was trying to leave. A few hours later, the nurse came in with a sitter in tow. "Why don't you go home, and we'll call you if there's a problem," she said.

This was sounding good, as I was exhausted. I seemed to live fairly exhausted, and when these peaks would hit, I was ready to crash. "Okay," I said, "but if the sitter needs to leave, call me—and give me twenty minutes to get here before she leaves."

It didn't happen. The sitter left. Mom tried to leave. And she fell. I guess hospitals are too busy to plan in advance. I didn't know till after the fall that there were "fall mats" that could have been on the floor. Much later I would learn about things like bed alarms, but I knew nothing at the time. Mom had a goose egg on her head—she didn't have a soft landing this time. However, it wasn't the fall that caused all the trouble. Mom wouldn't stay still for an MRI, so they gave her a sedative. It worked, but a little too well. It knocked her out for the test, and then it knocked her out for a lot longer. The downhill slide shocked me. Mom was semiconscious and hallucinating a lot.

"Look at all those loaves of bread up on the wall," Mom said one evening, pointing to something she was seeing very clearly. "Which one would you like?"

"I'll have wheat," I said, staring at the blank wall.

>>> Care Point 11 <<<

Don't leave an incapacitated person alone in the hospital. Get a caregiver or sitter. Get an extra bed or a chair for a family member to stay. Be an assertive, if not aggressive, advocate.

I'd never seen anything like this, and the idea of losing my mom was very real. The most frightening thing was the doctors. They didn't know my "real mom"—they knew only the elderly, somewhat delusional woman in front of them. "This isn't normal—she's not like this. Something is very wrong," I would tell any doctor who would listen. "Yes, she has Alzheimer's, but she's not at an advanced stage." I knew I was fighting a losing battle, and I knew they didn't have a clue about what to do. Apparently elderly people can be affected this way by sedatives. But Mom wasn't eating or drinking much. And she kept pulling her IVs out. They would wrap her up tightly, and Mom would patiently work her way out again.

We were in what is probably the biggest hospital in the DC area, with a reputation to match, and still Mom's care was cobbled together. The doctors were great. But neither the nurses nor I could quite master her care. We'd have a sitter. Then the sitter would suddenly have to leave, and I'd rush to get there. On some nights, they would move her bed to the hallway next to the nurses' station.

"Are you sure someone is always there?" I'd ask.

"Yes, I promise," a nurse would say. But on one of my visits, I noticed the area was empty. Maybe I should have thought about this myself, but it sure would have been nice if someone had said, "Get a private caregiver." It would have given me backup and placed someone in Mom's room whose only job was to watch Mom. Later I would do that.

>>> Care Point 12 <<<
Get help in the hospital. Friends may help, but pay for a private caregiver if necessary. Don't wear yourself down, and don't put your loved one at risk.

And then it was as though someone flipped a switch. It was early on a Saturday morning, and I called to check in with the sitter who should have been at Mom's bedside. But it was Mom's voice on the other end saying, "Hello?"

"Mom! Is that you?" I exclaimed.

"Well, whom were you expecting?" she quipped.

Immediately, I said, "Are you there alone?"

"Yes, they said they'll be back soon with breakfast."

Oh great. Mom was alone again. And now she was better. I needed to get there before she fell, and we started the process all over.

The change was dramatic. She was still pretty confused but lucid. My friend Rob joined me for a second visit later in the day, and we all talked and had a good time. It seemed very normal. The next day, I lugged my laptop and speakers to the hospital so we could "attend church" online—one of the benefits of going to a megachurch. Several nurses joined the caregiver and me as we went to church, with Lon Solomon, our pastor, blaring throughout our wing.

But it wasn't as though Mom was ready to go run a marathon. Late that night, a doctor said, "I'm going to go ahead and release your mother now, and you can go home."

"No, I don't want you to release her at this time of night," I said. "I don't feel comfortable taking her home to CARE-Assist without the daytime staff there."

"Ms. Nielsen," the doctor said sternly, "what your mother needs is for you to be a good daughter and be involved."

I stared at her, stunned. So stunned that I said nothing other than, "You cannot release her tonight." Our primary doctor had told me that they couldn't release someone without your agreement (up to a point, I suppose), and that knowledge came in handy. I went home and banged out a letter to the doctor, explaining that she was ignorant and naïve, and sharing the rest of my story with her. "You may be a good doctor," I wrote, "but if you have gotten to the point where you assume you know everything about your patients and their families, then perhaps it's time for you to try another profession." I was furious. How much more could one of me do? I stuck it in an envelope and went to bed.

"There is nothing wrong with your mom," a nice young doctor pronounced the next day.

"Then why does she keep falling?" I asked.

He was a little awkward as he said politely, "Well, she's old." Technically, he was right, but I wasn't convinced. This time I didn't protest when she was released. Really, I had this feeling that I needed to get her out of the hospital before something in the building killed her. As we left, I asked a nurse to promise to deliver my envelope to the doctor.

>>> Care Point 13 <<<
Think about when it's time to stop going to the hospital. Would in-home care be more appropriate?

When we arrived back at CARE-Assist, Mom was weak. Someone produced a wheel-chair, which was a good thing. We rode up in the elevator and into her new world. As the elevator doors shut behind us, an elderly woman walked up to us. She leaned in close and said loudly, with a venomous tone that I'll never forget, "Get out of my way, you stupid-looking fool."

I froze in horror. It seemed to go over Mom's head. But I couldn't get it out of mine. I looked back after we rushed past. "I can't protect my mom here," I thought, shaken. Here we were in this freshly renovated shared suite, and I knew we had to leave.

But something had happened. Somehow the hospital experience left Mom thinking really clearly. As she walked around her room picking up pictures, she held a picture of my father and said, "He's dead, isn't he?"

"Oh God," I prayed. "Help me hold it together." I was really good by now at changing the subject. It worked this time too, until Mom picked up a picture of her father. I thought my eyes were going to explode. Was I going to have to take the pictures away?

"He's dead too, isn't he?" Mom said tearfully.

I didn't have long to wonder, because I realized Mom was starting to sway in circles. Her feet weren't moving, but her torso seemed to be spiraling. I sprang up just in time to catch her and drag her to her bed. She was similar to how she'd been in the hospital. I'd seen "the look" again. She appeared to be semiconscious, but she was breathing. I called the office number for her PCP, Dr. Lessin, and he got on the phone right away.

"Drive back to the hospital, and ask for the same doctor who was overseeing her for this visit," he said. "They should just readmit you without going to the ER."

"Uh," I said awkwardly, "she said something that made me mad, and I left a scathing letter for her as we left."

He laughed and said, "Okay, call nine one one."

After calling, I ran to the desk and told them to prepare. Back we went to Fairfax Hospital, with me once again trailing behind an ambulance. As we had left, Karen said, "Julie, when you are at the hospital, ask them for information on hospice."

I stared at her quietly for a few seconds and said, "Okay." Was Mom nearing the end? I didn't know much about hospice. Or death.

To really understand my situation, you have to remember that all of this was happening on top of my hectic job. I was fairly successful at making both jobs work—my job as head of human resources and organizational development and my job as head of my mother. Shortly after Chris died, my CEO had said, "Take all the time you need, but when you are here, I need you here. You're going to have to get yourself together and *do* this."

He was right. How often had I said similar words when coaching employees? "You can have all of the good excuses in the world, but you still have a job to do." Many preretirement people will read this book, and to this group I say, "Be careful with your job." Don't lose it. If you think it's financially and physically hard taking care of a parent, try doing it in the fog of unemployment and uncertainty. I didn't intend to go there. And I knew my parents would want me employed and not shattered. I balanced the load by anticipating trouble. If I planned a business trip, I had a backup plan in case I had to skip it or return early. If there was any kind of event I had to coordinate, I had someone scheduled to step in on short notice. I did this for personal events too, although the number of those was dwindling as my life pulled me further and further away from any kind of a social life.

Care Concept #8: Keep Your Job...and Your Sanity

Few things in life are as important as caring for or protecting a loved one. But you must balance their lives and yours and draw boundaries. Learn to accept imperfection and do the best you can to get by. Your employer will most likely be supportive up to a point, but you still have a job to do, and your employer is not a charity. Do your job, and do it well. Force time into your schedule for yourself. Remember David Allen's book I mentioned earlier—*Getting Things Done*. It will help you with this balancing act.

If I needed any more confirmation that people thought Mom's situation was serious, I got it at the hospital late that night. Another one of the nice young doctors came to update me. They were "checking a few things."

"No more MRIs," I said.

"Definitely not," he agreed. "But I'm going to give you a form, and I want you to take it home and think about it."

I stared at the form and recognized it instantly. "Do Not Resuscitate Order" was written at the top. This was the form I would sign to tell people not to go to heroic measures to restart my mom's heart if it stopped.

"I'm signing it," I mumbled.

"No, take it home," he said.

"Look, my mother told me a hundred times what she wanted." I truly knew what to do—there was no doubt in my mind. My mother had hammered it into my head. I signed it, and it went in her file.

"Good night," he said. "I'm really sorry you're having to go through this alone." So was I. I went to the dark, empty cafeteria, sat down, put my head in my hands, and cried.

I like to keep quotes. I store them in a folder on my computer, noting where I saw them or who gave them to me. Leadership, life, and humor—they run the gamut. My favorite one came to me around this time, though I don't remember where I found it. It's from C. S. Lewis's book *The Silver Chair*. He wrote, "Crying is all right in its way while it lasts. But you have to stop sooner or later, and then you still have to decide what to do." How frequently this quote would pull me through. "Go ahead and fall apart, but then pull yourself together and get your job done," I would think. I had many opportunities in my life to put this to work. I lived in just-get-the-job-done mode.

Care Concept #9: Powers of Attorney and Advance Directives (DNRs)

You should contact an estate attorney and an elder-care consultant, even if you don't engage them. They can share more details on the subject of powers of attorney and advance directives. I hear story after story of several siblings being put in charge of decision-making—for medical and end-of-life decisions as well as financial ones. I had the sad benefit of being the only decision maker, which was hard and easy at the same time. Hard because I did it alone, but easy because I didn't need to debate anyone. Consider identifying one child as the primary decision maker, asking them to consult the others. A DNR is not what you may think. It does not preclude medical care; it simply indicates not to take heroic steps to restart a stopped heart. Learn more about them.

Out once again, we left the hospital. It was a beautiful day, and we stopped for gas. Mom seemed fine, and she jumped at the idea of having lunch—real food after hospital food. Our parking spot was across from the door to Jason's Deli, and I left Mom at the table while I went and ordered. We enjoyed lunch and our return to normalcy. We stood up and began to walk arm in arm toward the car. And then it happened. It was the look, and Mom wouldn't talk to me. We were in the middle of the street, and I put my hands on Mom's arms and said, "Mom, will you answer me? Are you okay?" She wasn't. I caught my mom once again. Cars were coming from both directions, but they stopped as they saw what was happening. A man ran out from the restaurant and said, "I'm an EMT, can I help?"

"Can you help me get my mom to the car?" I said quietly. He was big enough to mostly carry her, and he put her in the car seat. He whipped out his cell phone and started to dial 911. "No, that's okay," I said. "I'm going to drive her back to the hospital. She was just discharged." He looked at me like I was nuts at first, as in, "Lady, your mother is clearly in trouble." But then he looked at Mom and seemed to get it. I thanked him profusely as he walked away, and I noticed that there were several bystanders observing us. I smiled wanly and got in the car. At least when I was with Mom, I never failed to catch her.

I noticed a trend on this day. It was always when Mom stood up. Within minutes of her getting put in the car, she was fine. In the last incident at CARE-Assist, Mom had stood up from the wheelchair and a few minutes later collapsed. Now this time she had stood up from the table and collapsed. I thought about her other falls that I hadn't witnessed and wondered if they had happened the same way.

"I think I know the pattern," I said to the doctor and explained my theory. He agreed, and a short time later they would finally identify the problem. Mom had orthostatic hypotension, a blood-pressure issue where pressure is normal while sitting (which is typically what you are doing when blood pressure is measured), and it drops when one stands up. Mom was continually prone in the hospital, and no one ever thought to check her pressure while she was standing.

"We have a decision to make," the doctor said after it was all confirmed. "Your mother's blood pressure is on the high side when she is sitting or standing, which is why she takes meds for it. Then it's low when she stands."

"So," I picked up, "we have to choose between letting it be too high or too low?"

He smiled and said, "You hit it on the head." I knew pretty quickly what to do. She couldn't keep falling—breaking bones and being bruised and bloodied wasn't going to work. That meant we would need to live with an increased likelihood of stroke by raising her blood pressure all of the time so it wouldn't drop so low when she stood up.

It worked. Although I was always aware of the risk, Mom stopped falling. When we left the hospital this time, I knew it was the last. Barring a broken bone or something catastrophic, Mom would not be back.

Before leaving the hospital, I did as Karen at CARE-Assist had suggested: I met with hospice. Mom would qualify, and we would soon be in. I entered the phase where I knew Mom's death could be six months away—the technical definition of who gets into hospice.

CHAPTER 12

The Return Home

By this time, my decision to leave CARE-Assist and return to the condo was made. I kept going back and forth mentally, but I knew in my heart what I needed to do. Back at CARE-Assist after the last visit, I arranged for a caregiver from CARE-Home because Mom needed more assistance than CARE-Assist could provide. I did the calculation one evening. We were rushing through an annualized $250,000 per year. And we couldn't sustain it long, or the threat of running out of money would be immediate.

Care Concept #10: Parental Savings Accounts

Can your parents crank through $6,000 to $10,000 a month for three to five years? If they have this kind of savings, you just need to know where the money is and what their wishes are. But if they don't, you have some planning to do *now*. Your own savings may need to go toward your parents' care. Will you have enough?

One quarter of a million dollars. Much of what I am sharing in this book applies whether you are wealthy or not. My parents weren't wealthy, but they had planned. But I think even wealthy people would begin to struggle under those numbers at some point. My parents' planning ability had left me in the position to write checks for really big amounts for a limited time. It's just that the funds were dwindling, and fast. We have 401(k) accounts. We have savings accounts and mutual funds. But are we as a nation really saving for our parents' care? I don't think so. Some kids find it easy to stick their parents somewhere and walk away. I saw those some at CARE-Assist. But most of us can't—we were raised to go into battle for our parents. And this is the group that needs to be planning.

But that image of the woman who yelled at Mom lived in my memory and made me shudder. And the ring! Why did I have to have to keep my mother's ring? I gave notice and began making plans to have the condo carpeted and painted in advance of Mom's arrival.

We had made friends at CARE-Assist—Mom and I both. Most of them were residents, but we were fond of some of the employees too. I didn't like the idea of leaving Sue and her mom. Not too much later, they would leave as well. They too would pack up their camera and go, in search of the ideal-care situation. What would the residents do without us? Frankly, without me? I kept an eye out for a number of people, and I would sit and talk to many of them. They were beautiful. But in the end, I decided that I had only enough of me to worry about my mother. I was a crusader, but I had realized my limitations at saving the world.

This time, we had to upsize—we had gotten rid of so much that I had to borrow and buy a few more items. Back the movers came to pick up furniture and retrieve other items from my house. When I set Mom's camera up, this time in the condo, it didn't work—it hadn't survived the move. Remembering our family decision, I searched for a new one. This one came from New York, not Israel. I hoped Chris wouldn't mind. It was a different camera now, but I still remembered Mom's words: "We need to protect me." Two married friends, Phil and Barbara, lived in the building, and they became responsible for changing the camera card out when I needed it. I would call them when we were all leaving, and they would enter the condo and make the switch. It had been easier at CARE-Assist because Mom and I didn't need to be secretive, and we talked about the camera a lot—sometimes we'd joke and pretend we were putting on a show. But now there was a caregiver. I located the camera in the living room, where Mom would spend most of her time and where there was no legal expectation of privacy.

>>> Care Point 14 <<<
Check the laws for your state. They vary with regard to videotaping.

The place looked great when Mom walked in that first night. It smelled of fresh paint, and the next morning, it would be sunny and warm. Once again, Ruth and Pat had taken her out for the day. Once again, Ann and I went to work making it look just right.

I wondered if we would raise any flags at the Renaissance. After all, it was a hip place after the facelift it had received when it went condo—definitely not the typical place for seniors. But even after I submitted a form to get approval to have an additional lock installed, no flags went up. I'm sure it was a fire-code violation—the lock could be locked from the inside, helping ensure that Mom didn't go anywhere when a caregiver looked away or fell asleep. But I figured that the caregiver would always be there and would get them out in case of fire. I had locks installed on the sliding doors and the sliding windows after reading that people with Alzheimer's had fallen out of windows trying to escape. We would keep a low profile for quite a while to avoid the appearance of being a liability.

I also found a bed alarm, which would serve us well for years. It was a plastic strip that went under the sheet on the bed. As soon as there was no pressure from someone lying on it, the alarm went off. It was loud and obnoxious, but to be safe, I also purchased a baby monitor, which would carry the sound into the caregiver's room.

>>> Care Point 15 <<<
Most people with Alzheimer's are mobile. Bed alarms alert you to when they are on the move.

The condo was ideal for two people. When we purchased it, I had liked the idea of having the second bedroom for company. But now it was ideal for a caregiver. They would each have their own room and bathroom. In between was a kitchen, to the right as you entered, leading to a large living and dining area. Without much hesitation, I engaged CARE-Home in caregiving. They were advising me. We had a wonderful companion, Cindy, through them. It was natural that I would turn to them for the final piece—the actual caregiving. I had enough hesitation to interview three private caregivers. They were nice enough, and the cost would have been a little more than half of what I would be paying CARE-Home. But it seemed that I would be getting a lot more for that premium fee, which I ultimately elected to pay. They would do background checks and employment references. There would be backup when the primary caregiver went on vacation or was sick. They would do training. They would employ the person; I would employ the company. They would provide full service revolving around my mother and me.

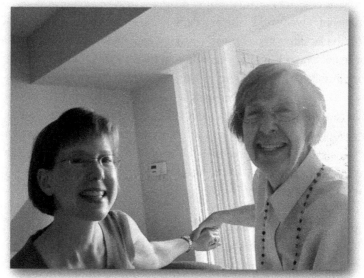

Goofing off in the condo

Susie was the first caregiver, and I liked her as soon as I met her. She was good with Mom despite her youth—she was quite young, perhaps twenty-four or so. She was from Ghana and loved Facebook. Although she was on her phone a lot, I could tell she took good care of Mom. I had let the CARE-Home people pick her, trusting them completely to make the best decision. I assumed they knew more than I did. And I also knew that options were limited. During her brief time with us, she would take weekend trips periodically. A backup caregiver would come in her place. This is how I first met Grace.

CHAPTER 13

Finding Grace (I)

liked her instantly. Grace was older than Susie by far—just a few years older than I. I had laughed when Susie told me about her over the phone. "She is an elderly woman," she said.

"Elderly?" I thought. "That could be nice. Someone to understand Mom better. But what if she isn't strong enough?" When I showed up that night on Grace's first stay, a woman close to my age opened the door. Later, when Susie returned, I said, "Susie, why did you tell me Grace was elderly?"

"She is!" Susie said with a quizzical look.

"She's my age...is that elderly?" I asked.

She laughed and said, "In Ghana, your elders are all elderly, no matter how old they are."

"That doesn't apply in this country," I said with a laugh, "so I'd be careful with those words."

One day my phone rang at work—not on the cell phone, so not a cause for alarm. "There is a little water on the floor in my bathroom," Susie said. After having her describe it, it didn't sound like an emergency. I'd go over after work and put my limited plumbing skills to work. But when I walked in, I was shocked. The water was a half an inch deep all over the bathroom, held back only by the threshold at the door. "Susie!"

I exclaimed, as I ran toward the toilet and reached for the shutoff. "This is *not* a little bit of water! You should have told me it was standing water." I was mindful still of the five floors below us. I noticed over our years with caregivers that they weren't quick to solve problems. I got the sense that in their countries, one tolerated problems.

If you go this route for care, don't rely on the caregiving company to train the caregivers. You need to know for yourself—however good the company is. My company, one with a stellar reputation, said they trained them, but I frequently saw things that made me question whether that was true. Looking back, I should have planned better. I would have trained on basic home maintenance (like turning off a toilet), fire prevention, and food safety. One day I was looking for a snack in the pantry and saw a partially used jar of spaghetti sauce.

"In Ghana we don't put things like that in the refrigerator," Susie had said.

"Well, in America, we do," I had said firmly.

>>> Care Point 16 <<<
You need to be the chief trainer, so make a plan. It's especially true with home care, but it also applies at a facility.

On a later visit, it was Grace, not CARE-Home, who told me that Susie wasn't coming back. She was supposed to be taking a two-week trip to Ghana. "Ju-lee," Grace said in her level, almost monotone voice, "Susie packed up her things. It's empty. I knew when I came here this time that she would not be back." I hadn't noticed because I rarely went into Susie room. That night Susie called and told me herself. Grace had been right.

"Are you looking for live-in work, Grace?" I asked.

"Yes, I am," she said happily. I e-mailed CARE-Home and told them the news. They agreed that Grace would be a good fit.

And so began the odd family that would last over three years. The entry of Grace into our lives seemed like such a blessing. I thought it probably was. Everyone said it was. I was the lucky one CARE-Home pointed to as an example. This trio of a genteel

Southern woman, her fiercely protective daughter, and a Ghanaian woman…we made quite the team. I laughed at how quizzical Dad and Chris would be if they could somehow walk back in the door and see how our family had changed. But a family we were. I called us Team Nielsen. And before long Mom and I were eating fried plantains, rice ball and chicken soup, and an assortment of other dishes that were new to us. But typically, Grace fixed traditional American food for Mom and Ghanaian food for herself.

Making My Cave

Not too long after this, I started "caving." No, not spelunking. More like nesting. I was creating my cave, knowing that I would retreat into it now, and then later as things got worse. My house—a three-story brick colonial townhome—was built around 1986, and it looked it. Back when I had bought the house in 1997, I was glum when I moved in and realized the house didn't look nearly as good as it had when my friend Audrey owned it. She had beautiful furniture, and my postcollege crate furniture just wasn't the same. Audrey was an older coworker at a company where I worked at the time. I had visited with her a few times and drove her to work on snowy days. I loved the house and had told her to tell me when she was ready to retire and sell it. I meant it, but I thought I had time. Then something made Audrey advance her schedule. I wasn't prepared either mentally or financially, but with Mom's cross-country advice, I had decided that this was my house. I stretched at the time, but after surviving on the edge financially for a couple of years, it turned out to be a great move. I wished so much that Dad could have seen it—I knew he would have been proud.

I would do little things to the house over the years but nothing large scale. During the time Mom was ill, taking care of my cave gave me solace. I would close the door and lock out the world. A few enhancements made it "me." I tried to show Mom a few times. "Hey, Mom, look, I put in a new kitchen floor." Mom would look at the ceiling and say it was beautiful. Chris would have had fun with the changes too—he loved working on my house as much as working on his. But there was no one to be proud, so it became even more my cave. It wasn't my family's home, even though family memories decorated it throughout. It was becoming my home. I spent the money carefully, though, knowing that my money would become Mom's money if we ran through hers.

Ken took on Chris's role in many ways. He had gotten me through the year after Chris's death. One winter day after an unusually large but beautiful snowstorm (when ultimately several feet of snow would be dumped on the DC area), I went out for a walk with Sasha. When I returned, water was gushing through the living room window. "Water…living room window…I'm trying to catch it with a bucket," I blurted out as Ken answered the phone. The beautiful snow that I loved was now melting and pouring in.

Ken was so much like Chris. No *hello* was required. His response was, "When I say go, run upstairs, rip down your shower curtain, get scissors and duct tape. Then run back to the phone. Now *go!*" I'm a single woman who loves Home Depot and tools, and I actually had duct tape. We crafted a gutter to catch most of the water. Each time I would empty the bucket, I'd wonder what I would do without him. The cave was secure, and I would have the problem fixed later.

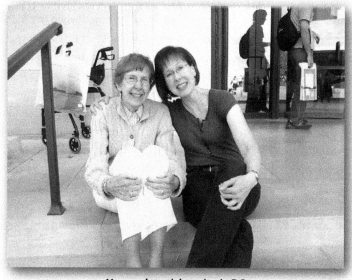

Mom and me sightseeing in DC

CHAPTER 14

Assisted Living, Part II

The only obvious thing we needed to do was get Grace to lower her voice. It seemed to me that Africans are loud, boisterous people. They seem happy and outgoing. But Mom was a Southern gentlewoman. Loud noises and loud voices bothered her. And Grace was loud. That was probably the only thing that worried me about her early on. Cindy was still Mom's companion and took her out to lunch, grocery shopping, and walking at the mall. She was part of the team too—I adored her and her family. I hadn't met her college-aged kids in person, but she, her husband, Mom, and I had gone out on more than one occasion and had a great time. Cindy was a rock, always calm and steady. I'm steady, but not always calm. So she balanced me.

Grace and Mom became well known at the Renaissance. Mom liked to walk—a lot. They would walk the hallways and sit in the lobby to people watch. We were back under the eyes of the security staff, and we knew all of them. They frequently gave me reports on what was going on. I always had trouble walking as slowly as Mom walked. It was so slow I couldn't quite get my legs to work that way. But Grace had no trouble. They lumbered along like a ship, with Grace in command.

Grace never seemed to worry. So I did all the worrying for both of us. In times of crisis, she got calm and kept on lumbering. I went into director mode and told everyone what to do. I guess the combination worked well. I remember what Chris's wife had said after he died: "Why do you have to direct everything?" I thought to myself in response, "I'm a director." And I was. I couldn't do much about it.

>>> Care Point 17 <<<
Help caregivers generate ideas for activities—for example, care for plants, use tools, sort fabrics, create photo albums, or visit a Michael's store.

With Karen's plea in mind, my plan was to have a caregiver who would also be the social director. CARE-Home tried to help come up with activities, but they never stuck with it. So the day revolved around walks and television. I had hoped they would do more, and I wished Mom could even help more with household chores, like laundry. But I decided that the slow pace and limited activities would have to do.

I noticed early on that Grace didn't take enough breaks. I voiced my concern to a manager at CARE-Home, who said, "This is what they do, Julie; they are here to make money, and some of them don't have anywhere to go home to." Grudgingly, I agreed we would not force more frequent breaks. But when Grace would go away, it rarely went well. It was a familiar routine. She would leave on a Friday morning. I would go over Friday night to meet the backup caregiver and make sure she was clear on the instructions. I would know in ten minutes if the person was good or not. I could tell by the instructions they retained, my ability to understand them, and by how they treated Mom. Those who treated her like a child were a disaster—Mom would get furious and attempt to leave, triggering a weekend-long battle.

>>> Care Point 18 <<<
If using a caregiver, require breaks. Alzheimer's patients can be tedious at best—and abusive at worst. They wear you down.

One night I went over for one of these checks. A pleasant but exasperated-looking young woman greeted me at the door with the phone in her hand. I heard her say to her manager, "I'll call you back—the daughter is here." She hung up and addressed me. "Your mother threw her cereal at me and then tried to hit me with a pillow," she said.

"Not good," I thought. Mom wouldn't do that unless something was terribly wrong. I even wondered if the woman was lying. But the fact that her front was wet indicated she was telling the truth. Not to mention the fact that Mom was standing in the living room with a pillow raised above her head when I walked in to see her.

"Oh, hi!" she exclaimed as I walked in. "I don't like her."

"I can tell." I smiled. I was pretty good at getting these situations toned down, and we always survived.

I never really felt like the backup caregivers meant any harm to Mom. Instead, they were just ill equipped. Grace would know too—she required only ten minutes to determine their ability to handle Mom. One weekend I noticed an unexplained bruise on Mom's arm. It was enough for me to ask Phil and Barbara to pull the camera card. Sure enough, within minutes of Grace leaving, Mom had fallen. It looked like a trip. Violating what we always called our number-one rule, the weekend caregiver pulled Mom up. The rule was to let her sit on the floor and to call me. If I couldn't get there in minutes, I would be the one to call nine one one. When I questioned her, the caregiver never let on that there had been a fall. Yet another e-mail would go to CARE-Home saying, "She can't come back." I never let on that we had a camera, so I did not provide specifics. The overriding issue I saw was simply honesty—people not telling the truth about what was actually happening.

Is This It?

Maybe everyone with a loved one who is dying goes through this. But I frequently wondered how it would happen. What would I be doing when Mom died? Sleeping? Working? Would I be with her? Would I make it over in time to say good-bye? It was with that backdrop that I answered the phone at two o'clock one morning. The nighttime phone calls always had me up and moving quickly. I was ready to move fast at a moment's notice. "Your mother fell and she isn't breathing," Grace yelled into the phone.

I was on my feet and pulling sweats on over my pajamas as I ran. "Is there blood? What happened?" I said breathlessly as I headed down the stairs.

"She's not breathing, she's not breathing," was all I could hear.

"This is it," I thought. "If she's not breathing now, she won't be breathing when I get there."

I could get to Mom's fast anytime, but at two in the morning, I was like lightning. The entry gates were open, as they typically were for an emergency. And I could see the ambulance at the front entrance. Why had Grace waited to call me? I clearly didn't get quick notice. I'm not sure my car had come to a complete stop before I was out and running. A police officer walked toward me, and I seem to recall him saying, "Stop," but I was a woman on a mission. I bolted past reception and into a waiting elevator. "Come on," I said as I pounded the sixth-floor button. Out I ran before the doors could fully open. I was running at breakneck speed, and I was breathing so hard that I couldn't hear what the man at Mom's door was saying. When I clearly didn't hear him, he stepped fully into the hallway and waved his arms—possibly because the odds were good I was about to mow him down. I slowed down just enough to hear him yell, "Alert and conscious! Your mom is alert and conscious!" I was panting and couldn't stand up straight. "I asked the police officer downstairs to tell you, so I don't know how he missed you."

"He tried to stop me," I panted sheepishly.

"Why don't you wait out here while we check her out," an EMT said.

Grace and I had a few minutes to talk, and she was near tears. "It was awful, Julie. I was so scared. And I forgot and called nine one one instead of you."

"What was the worst part?" I asked.

I had to work hard to hide a laugh when Grace said, "They had me give her CPR. It was hard to do because your mom was trying to get away from me."

"Grace," I said, "the next time you do CPR on someone, you might want to make sure they aren't trying to get away from you."

The EMTs were furious when they realized that there was a DNR in place. I underscored to Grace how we had to honor Mom's wishes. She was horrified when I told her how, without it, Mom could have a heart attack and doctors might end up breaking her ribs trying to save her.

We heard Mom yell from the bedroom, and an EMT yelled, "Owwwww." Mom was mad and probably scared and had landed a kick. "Ms. Nielsen, maybe you should come in now."

I got down on the floor and explained what was going on to her. I could tell she was fine, and like usual, my voice calmed her down. They got her up and put her back in bed. I think what really happened was that Mom got out of bed and fell. Grace heard the alarm and came running, and Mom lay on the floor with her eyes closed. In Grace's mind, I would learn, someone lying on the floor was the same as someone lying on the floor not breathing. I explained the difference, and we drilled on possible responses many times over the coming months.

Even CARE-Home didn't fully grasp the DNR concept. They thought it meant care would be denied to someone in need. That was crazy—no medical professional would deny care. It meant only that heroic measures would not be taken to restart a stopped heart.

Grace's first Christmas with us as a full-time caregiver was the last trip Mom and I took. "Ju-lee," Grace said as she called me, "I don't think that you can do it."

Now I had been issued a challenge. "I can do this, Grace," I said confidently. She knew that a lot had changed since I'd taken care of my mom twenty-four-seven. I was good at fulfilling what my role had become—not at living with her.

Grace was right. It was rough. The hotel staff helped me muddle through, but let's just say it was not pleasant, and it definitely wasn't a vacation. Still, Mom and I enjoyed walking along the quaint streets of the Revolutionary War town and shopping. "Let's buy something fun to bring home," I said. Mom picked out a brightly colored ceramic heart with the word "laugh" on it. How like my mom. I knew it would serve as a reminder for me, and it does today. Driving the hour and a half home, I knew it was our last trip.

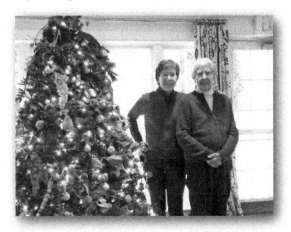

Mom and me in St. Michaels, Maryland, for Christmas

The following Christmas we would turn St. Michaels into a day trip, driving down late morning, enjoying dinner at the Inn at Perry Cabin, and then driving back home. Grace joined us, and it was fun seeing her enjoyment of the five-star restaurant. Mom and Dad are to blame for my enjoyment of nice restaurants. And nothing made me happier than pampering Mom.

The next Christmas we would stick closer to home. Mom and I had a nice break-fast at the Ritz Carlton, and then Grace joined us for dinner late that afternoon. It was a beautiful day even though we didn't travel anywhere. At breakfast that day, it was so good to see glimpses of my old Mom. An interesting (and apparently single) man sat next to us, and we chatted during our meal. At one point, Mom said loudly, "Don't let him get away." I was fairly certain he heard, and I had to laugh. Later, as he helped Mom put her coat on to leave, Mom said, "You'd better run while you can." He and I both howled. Nothing came of it, but Mom sure tried hard. She knew exactly what was going on.

That's how Christmases went.

Headed to church one Sunday, traffic came to a sudden stop, and I had to brake hard. The driver of a Mustang behind us noticed too late. That noise an accident makes is awful. The bang and the crunching metal. Luckily, it was mostly his metal that was doing the crunching. We were in my Honda CR-V, and his car was "submarining" as he braked to avoid us. The impact left his shorter car up under my taller SUV. Mom and I both yelled.

"What happened?" Mom exclaimed.

"We just got hit. Are you okay?" I said anxiously.

"I feel fine," Mom said. "I'll handle this. You stay here."

"No!" I shouted as I made sure her door was locked. I smiled. "I'll take this, and *you* stay here." We were on a busy street, and impatient people were lining up behind us.

Luckily no one was injured, and several people stopped to see if we were okay. I was shaken, though. The car was drivable, since the Mustang just damaged the bumper and the exhaust system as it went up under us. So after getting the driver's information, we turned around and went back to my house. Mom and I sat in the den, and I called the insurance company to report the claim. At first, Mom sat patiently next to me as I talked. But then she blurted out, "Why are you telling people we had an accident when we didn't?"

"Shhhhh!" I hissed, covering the phone. "Mom, we *did* have an accident."

"No, we didn't," she said, looking irritated. I decided it was a good thing I hadn't called the police. What if Mom had said the same thing to them? It could have gotten complicated. I called Grace, who panicked at the idea of an accident. Then we all did what the Nielsen women do under stress: we went to lunch.

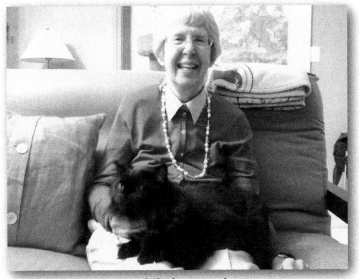

Mom and Charlotte at my house

Looking for Monsters

A few things worried me, and they worried Mom's friends as well. Mom didn't want to go home when she had been out. "That woman thinks she can boss me around in my own home," Mom had told Barbara and John. And it nagged at me that Mom always thought Grace and the backups were men. I think it was their dark skin, short hair, and, frequently, large size. And I was worried about the backup caregivers, who did not seem to be well trained.

"She was crazy," Grace would say after a less-than-good one.

"Why didn't you tell me that before you left?" I'd say. I would e-mail CARE-Home with updates or to say certain caregivers couldn't return. One day, Grace told me that I could never tell them that she and I talked about care quality.

"Be careful with all those e-mails you send," she had said. "Don't get me in trouble." But our opinions always aligned.

At a routine visit to a doctor who I had seen for years and who had seen Mom when she first moved back, I said, "Maybe I should bring Mom back in just to be safe... so you could check her out."

"Julie," said the doctor, whom I admired greatly, "don't go looking for monsters."
I decided he was right. I would see Grace on the camera too when I would check on the backup caregivers. In my short glimpses of life at Mom's, things seemed normal. I would tell others in various situations over the years, "Don't go looking for monsters."

CHAPTER 15

Fire

can look back and identify many times where I was so over my head. Sometimes, I felt like I could feel myself dying, little by little, from the stress. Like the stress was eating me little by little. Clearly Chris's death and the emotional and physical aftermath was the top example of this. But there was a close second.

For a few weeks the following winter, the fire alarm had been going off at the Renaissance. It was getting irritating for everyone who lived there, but I knew better than to always assume they were false alarms. I always slid into action just to be safe. Then in April, at the end of a particularly rough day, I fell into bed. I remember praying, "Please give me a good night's rest. Help me wake up strong again." I don't recall why now, but I was running on fumes.

That was eleven o'clock. At two, the phone jolted me awake. There was noise on the line, and then I heard Grace's voice. "Fire alarm," she said, and then there were only garbled words.

"Grace, is it just the alarm, or do you smell smoke?" I yelled into the phone.

More garble. And then Grace's voice broke through. "There is fire." The line went dead.

I pulled on sweats and shoes while running and made the familiar bolt for my car. The Renaissance was a big brick building. How could it burn? But as I hit the street next to mine that leads to the Renaissance, I stopped. I was attempting to join a long line of fire trucks. "Oh God," I thought. "This is for real."

Ken always says that if he's ever in a high-speed car chase again, he wants me driving. I learned how to drive on Washington's Beltway, so jumping in between fire trucks was nothing. I had contemplated running instead, but I jumped between trucks when I saw a gap. As soon as I was inside the gates, I ditched my car and ran. People in pajamas were everywhere, with children crying and dogs barking. I passed cats in crates and people on cell phones—and what appeared to be every fire truck in Fairfax County. It was a big complex, with many people who might need saving. I was in shock as I hit the lobby. The smoke was thick, but people were still in it, taking shelter from a chilly rain. I stopped at the reception desk and said frantically to the guard, "Have you seen Grace and my mom?"

He looked stricken. "Oh no. I forgot. Let me get a fireman."

No time. I ran toward the left stairway that would be closer to mom's side of the building. The building was the shape of a Y, but I was a little turned around in all the chaos. A fireman tried to stop me, and I yelled, "Disabled mom in apartment six fifteen" as I ran by him. I'm not a good runner, but I was doing really well on adrenaline, bounding up the stairs after already having run across the large parking lot. But as I crossed the third-floor landing, my phone rang. I slowed enough to grab it and saw Grace's number.

"We're at the back of the building," Grace yelled. They weren't far away, and I left the stairwell and headed toward the rear door in the darkened hallway. The slope of the grounds provides for ground exits on the first, second, and third floors, and Mom and Grace had made it down from six to three before following a crowd out the rear door.

The first thing I noticed when I saw them was that Mom was fully dressed, not in her pajamas like everyone else. I closed my eyes and thought, "I never talked to Grace about this. I never gave her a fire plan." Clearly CARE-Home hadn't either. How could I, the one responsible for my organization's crisis-management plan, *not* have a plan for my own mother? I would tell Grace later not to get dressed before evacuating next time. We trudged in the chilly night back around to the lobby, where they were letting people sit. Despite the smoke, no one could see flames. We all assumed it was a small mishap, and we waited for the all-clear sign from fire officials. Then word got around: there had been an explosion in the fifth-floor electrical room. "Let's wait a little while longer," I said. We met a wonderful woman named Connie, who was sitting in a chair with a cane by her side. But overall, no one said much. Kids slept, and the rest of us just sat and breathed the smoky air.

The training plan I referred to earlier should include crisis planning. What do you do if there's a fire? Living in DC, I had to ask this one: "What if there is a terror attack?" We decided later that we would do what's called *sheltering in place* in case of another fire. No trying to carry Mom down the stairs and risking injuring her. Grace knew to call nine one one, tell them she and Mom were in the unit and couldn't leave, and go out on the balcony if necessary. I thought how funny it was that Mom's fear of being past the reach of the fire trucks was now helpful. Later I called the county and asked if they could make a note in the Renaissance file that there was a disabled person in Unit 615. They noted it, but I don't think I would have relied on that alone. I told Grace later, "If there were a terror attack, just know I'm making my way to you. Leave only if the building is damaged."

About four o'clock, the Red Cross showed up to start assisting residents. "Okay, we're done," I said. I walked over to Connie and said, "Connie, you need to come home with us. I don't want to leave you here."

"Oh no, I'll be fine. I'm sure they'll let us up soon," she said. I pushed, but she held firm.

"Then take my cell phone number, and call if you need me." We made our way around the fire trucks and back to my car, back to my house, and upstairs. We got Mom into bed and put an air mattress on the floor so Grace could block Mom's exit—and access to the stairs. I climbed back into bed around five and lay there for just seconds, pondering how things could go so wrong. And then the phone rang. It was Connie.

"I think you'd better come and get me. They are saying it's a big problem."

"I'll be right there," I sighed. Back I went, this time driving in figure eights around the trucks. Now I was in my pajamas and said, "Hello again" as I passed the firefighters. There was Connie. I had told Grace I was leaving, but there wasn't a sound when Connie and I returned. I had locked the pets (now three cats with the addition of Charlotte, plus Sasha) in the den. I set up another bed for Connie, and we all slept for a few hours.

You can only sleep for so long when you are on a dog-walking schedule. And something was going on at work that would require me to go in that afternoon. After a little sleep, I got up to make breakfast for my houseguests. The conversation was great, and I enjoyed listening as I got everything ready. But I looked at myself in the glass of my kitchen cabinet and thought, "How on earth did I get here? We've added someone from another country to the family, there's a stranger at my kitchen table, and they are all talking as though it's all very normal." It was almost funny, but not quite. I called Cindy for backup. She would take Connie to her friend's house. Before going to work, I drove to the Renaissance. The sign at the desk said, "Building has been closed—no power for two weeks." My heart sank. Mom couldn't handle my stairs well, and there was little room for her to walk around. This was going to be tough.

I headed to work, feeling pretty lousy in light of the events the previous night. Work was unremarkable, with a few people saying they had heard about the fire on the news. That evening I called up the stairs, "I'm home! I'm going to walk Sasha." Grace was cooking dinner, and it smelled great—a nice benefit of having her at my house. But something else didn't smell quite right. I opened the door to the den and was hit with an awful stench.

I don't know what Sasha had eaten. And I don't know how a fifty-pound dog could dispense out of both ends as much as she had. Half of the den was covered. Even now I can remember it clearly—twenty or thirty "piles" that she'd then walked in. The always-immaculate cats were perched up high at various locations. I was beaten down. That night, with Mom in bed, Grace and I spent hours on our hands and knees cleaning up the mess. "Ju-lee," Grace said, "it will get better." I wasn't so sure.

>>> Care Point 19 <<<
When life is hard, all of the bad events seem worse and more numerous. Keep your focus on the big picture.

And Sasha wasn't even done yet. Whatever she had wasn't going away, and it kept happening. It would last almost a week. So into the kitchen she went, locked in so I could clean up the mess from the floor and not the carpet. This cut Mom's walking room further, and she did not appreciate being blocked by baby gates that were now "Mom gates" as well.

The next morning, a Saturday, I drove back to the Renaissance to see if there was any good news. There wasn't. In fact, it had grown worse. It was now going to be a month, and the fire marshal had declared the building uninhabitable. But we were not barred from accessing it, so at least we could get things out of Mom's unit. I had already cleared the refrigerator the morning before, and now I brought other items over.

"Are you regretting moving your mom from CARE-Assist?" someone asked me as we chatted in the lobby.

"No," I said emphatically. Despite the current nightmare, it was still better.

Okay, time for a new plan. I had managed to let Saturday slip away, and now it was Sunday morning. I could think of two options: a furnished apartment or a temporary stay back at CARE-Assist. I went to both and looked at options. At the tall, beautiful apartment complex called Fairfax Towers not even a mile behind my house, they hadn't heard about the fire. I knew other residents would be close behind me, and I didn't have much time. CARE-Assist (another one nearby—not the one we had left) had plenty of room, but Mom couldn't come unless she had a TB test, which would take a couple of days. But they would let Grace stay with her.

I called Ann and said, "Help...we're in trouble and I need to make a decision." I was so tired that I couldn't think clearly.

Ann listened to the options and said, "Done. We're going to Fairfax Towers. And we'll do it now—you can't go into another week the way you are." She could see I was barely holding on. I was always the capable one who knew what to do, and I was losing my grip now. But then she said the words that she had said before and that meant so much: "I'm on my way." It's good to have friends who will step in and make decisions for you when you can't do it yourself.

When Ann and I hung up, there was one problem: I hadn't signed the lease. "I want the one-bedroom unit," I told the rental agent hurriedly. My thinking was that two bedrooms were risky—I needed Grace to block the door with some sort of bed. In the end, she would wind up pulling the sofa bed in front of Mom's doorway.

"I'm sorry," the manager said. "It's too late for a lease today, and it has to be approved." I don't know if she heard the desperation in my voice or if she remembered my description of my mother, as I'd made sure she knew that Alzheimer's was in the picture. But the next thing out of her mouth was, "I have to walk out the door at five. I'll have everything ready."

It was 4:45 p.m., and I was close by. As I ran by the living room on my way down two flights of stairs, I attempted to say calmly to Grace and Mom, "Girls, we're moving to the apartment tonight, so get ready."

"Stop!" Mom yelled.

I still followed my mom's instructions to the letter, and I froze. "What?" I asked.

"You can't be seven," she said.

"Forty-five and not too happy about it," I said.

"Oh, phew," was her response. "If you were seven, I didn't know how you'd be able to handle all this."

I laughed hard as I ran the rest of the way down and jumped in the car. It was good to laugh. Mom was beginning to step back in time, and I saw it with comments like this. But the thought of being seven and not having to worry about anything sounded pretty good.

As promised, the woman had everything laid out on the table. "Thanks," I panted as I sat down. I signed fast, never reading the documents—this time that would not turn out to be a problem, but I don't recommend hurrying on legal documents. She put the keys in my hand, and we were both out the door. Ann was sitting in the driveway when I pulled up. We loaded up the cars with items from my house and the condo, with barely enough room for people, and then unpacked at the Towers.

That night, I climbed into bed and enjoyed the silence of my own home. There would be no phone calls in the middle of the night.

CHAPTER 16

Routine Living

n the end, it took only fifteen days to get power restored to the building. Insurance covered everything—except my sanity. We reversed the plan and got Mom moved back in, and life moved on.

Sitting in church one Sunday, I wondered who would be preaching in the absence of our regular pastor. It was a man named Dale, and I hadn't heard of him before. Ten minutes after he started talking, I knew whom I would ask to conduct Mom's funeral when the time came. Dale was—somehow—an active-duty DC police detective as well as a pastor at the church. The police factor wasn't what made me pick him. It was that any detective, even though I had never met him face-to-face, had to understand real life. My real life wasn't neat and clean. It was pretty rough around the edges, and I figured Dale—as someone not always in the church building itself—would understand that.

That wasn't the only time I thought about Mom's funeral. Ways I could capture the essence of my mother would frequently appear in my brain. I created an electronic file called "What I Will Say," and I would make notes in it periodically. I knew that when the day finally came, I wouldn't remember anything without notes. I asked Pat if she thought that was weird, and she said no; she had had thoughts like that too before her dad died. That made me feel better.

I also decided I should be prepared for the logistics of death. Jennie did a survey of funeral homes for me, narrowing the list to three. Then we dropped it to two, and then one. After a visit, the decision was made and would not consume emotional real estate in the future. This was another example of a gift. She did the footwork and made something happen.

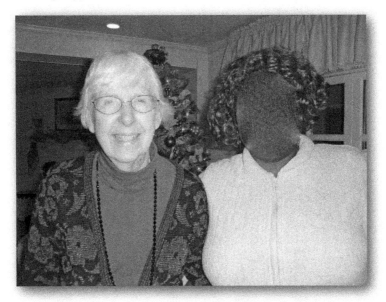

Grace and Mom at Christmas dinner in St. Michaels, the year after our last overnight trip

I feel smarter culturally from knowing Grace. She was not educated as far as I know, but she was still capable. We talked a lot, and I counted her as a friend, not just a caregiver. But I would never trust anyone 100 percent with my mother, not even her, and would leave the camera running as we had decided. I wasn't looking for monsters—just being vigilant.

I treated Grace the way I knew Mom would have treated her. She joined us at the Kennedy Center on one occasion and frequently joined us for nice meals. I bought her clothing, gifts, and other things she needed. She cried when I brought her a winter coat one cold winter. The Nielsen Team outings were always punctuated by laughter. Sometimes it was Grace and me laughing at a joke or teasing one another. Sometimes Mom started it. Frequently, Mom would get tickled at something only she understood and would go to pieces laughing. This would make Grace and me go to pieces as well. I knew how to appreciate these times.

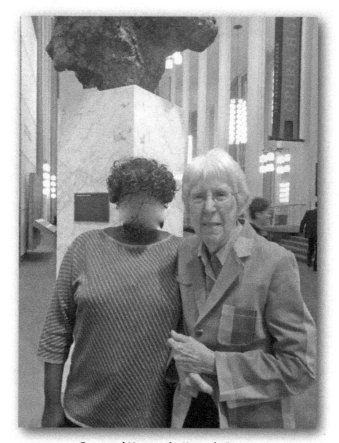

Grace and Mom at the Kennedy Center

"Who got shot?" Mom asked as I rushed into her bedroom one day in midmorning, after hurrying home from work. Grace had called me in a panic. There was blood everywhere, including Mom's head and her blouse. It was good she had me laughing, because the picture looked pretty grim. According to Grace, Mom had tipped backward, lost her balance, and hit her head on the doorframe as she went down. Per our rule, Mom was still sitting on the floor, leaning up against the wall and looking at a magazine. But I had a clear view of the risks of returning to the hospital now. The odds of a head injury were low. We'd just go to urgent care.

The cut wasn't that big, and about six staples took care of it.

"Does this hurt?" the doctor asked Mom as she started with the first staple.

"No," Mom replied. She winced a few times but didn't need a local anesthetic, which could have been more painful than the staples.

"Some people can handle it," the doctor said, but I thought about how other times of pain had seemed to go right over Mom's head. Grace was an expert on carpet cleanup by now, and the blood was completely gone the next time I went over.

Picture the best family you can imagine—parents who rarely make mistakes, adoring children—and you pretty much have my family. I used to say that we were like the *Father Knows Best* family, recalling reruns of a show that was old even when I was little. But no one can make the connection now. So when Mom popped out with "Go to hell" as she glared at me over her iced tea, I was stunned. There had been no yelling in my house, and little anger. If there was anger, it was the kind that got handled. And never—never—would anyone get cursed at.

Grace, Mom, and I were at a restaurant for my birthday lunch, and as we ate bread and waited for our food, I caught Mom as she was about to eat the plastic butter container. I lunged for it and said, "Don't eat that!" which prompted the "go to hell."

"Mom," I said dejectedly, "I just didn't want you to eat plastic."

"Well, don't tell me what to do like that," she snapped angrily.

I was hurt, and it was my birthday. "Ju-lee," Grace said, "your mother didn't tell you to go to hell, the Alzheimer's told you to go to hell." She was chuckling, which irritated me at first. But I shook my head and laughed. She was right. I frequently called her "Amazing Grace," and she would beam.

I became filled with worry each time Grace went away. The problems with backup caregivers were increasing. There was nothing catastrophic; they simply didn't understand how to treat an elderly woman like my mom. And they clearly didn't have enough training. They shouted (thinking she couldn't hear) and talked way too fast in their heavy accents. On one occasion, a caregiver called me for assistance. It was one I had concerns about already, based on my introduction to her the night before. I could hear raised voices as soon as I entered Mom's unit. She and Mom were in the bathroom, with the caregiver trying to help. I took the opportunity to quickly slip the camera card out of the camera and into my pocket unnoticed, and I headed toward them. But as I did, what I heard was awful.

"Get out of here before I call the police," Mom was shouting.

"I love you, I love you," the caregiver shouted back.

I was furious. I knew that Mom thought she was being attacked. She was in the bathroom with her pants down, and a stranger who she thought was a man was telling her "I love you." I knew the caregiver was trying to calm Mom down, but she didn't understand how horribly out of line her words were.

Upon her return Grace said, "I could see it right away."

"I could too," I agreed, "but just in case, you have to tell me when you have these concerns."

"They told me not to talk to you about things," she said.

I was troubled by this—the second time Grace had been told to be quiet. Was CARE-Home really more worried about the caregivers than my mother? Or was Grace misunderstanding them? At the time, I decided it was a little of both. I could see how they, as a business, might say, "Stay out of this employment discussion," but that was different from what Grace had said. But they kept telling me I had the ideal caregiving situation. We all liked Grace and just had to survive her weaknesses and her breaks.

Pat, who I mentioned before and is one of my closest friends, was a frequent visitor. The fact that she was retired allowed her to pitch in frequently over the years. She called me at work one day and said, "I left Hailey at your mom's for a while today. Do you know what they were doing when I left?"

Hailey is Pat's granddaughter, then eleven years old. "What?" I asked curiously.

"They were playing with their dolls."

That was a sweet picture. Most kids would have found this odd and probably scary. But Hailey was so adaptable—if Grandbet had a doll, she would just bring one over too. She cared deeply about my mom and had been brave and loving, as her great-grandfather had died the week before Chris.

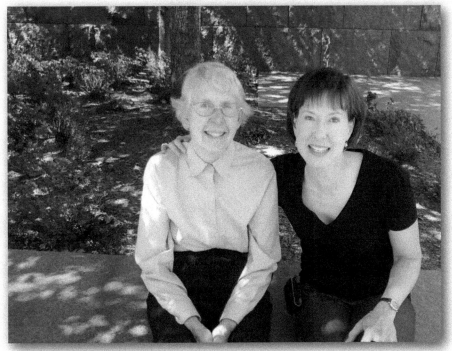

We kept up our visits downtown, this time at the Roosevelt Memorial.

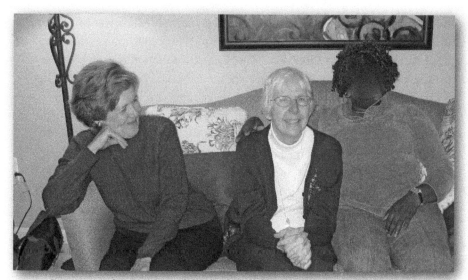

Pat, Mom, and Grace on Mom's last birthday. The Ritz Carlton in Tysons, Virginia, sent afternoon tea to us when it was too hard for Mom to go there.

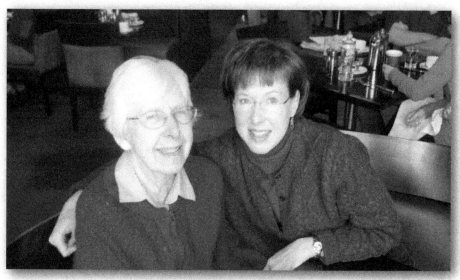

Before leaving for St. Michaels

Early in my life, I had it all together. I was a classic career woman, rolling out of college in the mid-1980s and landing one good job after another. Many times people said things like, "You are the most mentally stable person I know." Over these years, I would see my resolve and my abilities tested. Many nights I wondered how mentally stable I truly was. I learned that I was in much better shape when I had data—when I knew what my next steps would be. Planning ahead was invaluable. Before Jennie's father had died, we spent a Saturday looking at other assisted-living and nursing home options—just in case. And we came home depressed. It was the nursing homes that had me down, and I resolved that I could never let Mom get out of assisted living. I had to make sure the money lasted.

>>> Care Point 20 <<<
Don't plan for today. Plan for the end and for how you'll get there.

Month after month of challenges—some routine and some crushing—pummeled me, forcing me to be more realistic. And forcing me to learn what was really important. In the spring of 2012, a fairly large earthquake struck the DC area. Like most others, I was terribly frightened by it. My sixth-floor office swayed, shook, and rattled, and I decided that this was how I was going to die. Under my brick building. I didn't die. But a defining moment waited for me at home. ADT had called to alert me that the alarm was going off—like most other alarms in the area, so I wasn't overly concerned. Something had fallen off a wall and triggered the glass-break sensors, I was sure.

Maybe it was the fact that my townhome is an end unit. Or maybe it was just some freak of nature. But I was wrong. Much more awaited me. Lamps had been thrown off their tables. Drywall cracks appeared in most rooms. There was no structural damage, but I stood in the dining room, stunned, and stared at the family china cabinet. It had nearly gone over, dumping many items to the floor before tipping back toward its wall. The shaking caused miniexplosions of fine china on the inside, and most things that had left the cabinet were in pieces on the floor. I remembered when the movers had pulled it into the dining room after having to hoist it over my deck because of its large size. They told me, "Ms. Nielsen, you really should use the earthquake hooks that are on top, because this thing is huge." I had made a note to attach them one day. But an earthquake in Virginia? That was way down the list.

My grandmother's china, situated on the right side of the cabinet, survived—I was thankful for that. But a little set of yellow, black, and white china that Mom had collected over the years, situated on the left side, was almost completely destroyed.

"Do you want to keep the pieces?" my friend Margaret said when she arrived to help. Tears were streaming down my face and mixing with broken and powdered china. It was beyond hope. I was having trouble finding any hope at all. "You might be able to replace them if you search for their brands on the Internet," she said, trying to be helpful.

I fingered the pretty shards. They were finished. But I wasn't crying just for the shattered china. Everything was shattering. Life was shattering. There on my knees, I told myself that things were just things. Learning this was meaningful, because it freed me from worrying about other "things." My mom wasn't in a little shattered espresso cup or broken china egg holder. Mom was up the street, and I had a job to do.

How fickle nature is. I had called Grace and Mom from work as soon as the phone lines began opening up. Grace was frightened, but Mom didn't notice anything. The twelve-story building shook but sustained no damage. I think I worried a lot less after that day.

———

It's good to have talented friends. One of them is Wei, who says she's an amateur photographer but is as good as any professional I've seen. On a Sunday afternoon, Wei joined Mom and me at my house. She gave me another one of those priceless gifts—creative and beautiful. She took photo after photo of Mom and me. I knew as we were doing it that we were creating a picture memorial. There is something else I wish I had done: capture my mom on video back when she was more herself, and even later. Sometimes I struggle to hear my father's voice. I last heard it so long ago. But I remember his laugh. I can hear Chris's voice saying, "Mornin'," when he would come down in the early morning when he was visiting me or I was visiting him. Coffee time, while the kids were asleep, was our time.

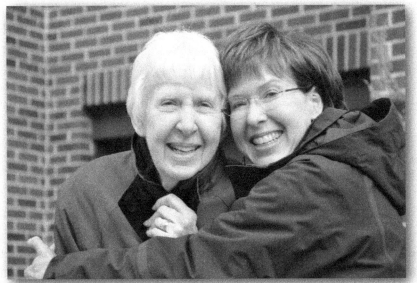

One of Wei's pictures outside; my favorite is on the cover of this book.

They Can't Mean Washington, DC

I had never heard of a derecho before. I don't think anyone in Washington had. But on a Friday summer night later that year, I noticed storm clouds as I drove home from getting a haircut. I flipped on the television while I was eating a late dinner. I'm not a Weather Channel watcher, but I stopped on it to hear them talk about a crazy storm. They mentioned Washington. "That has to be Washington state," I thought. There had been no storm warnings, and no alerts were coming over my iPhone. I usually received at least five alerts for what could sometimes be minor weather events. But not this time. I called Rick to check in, and he was rattled—four hours away.

"This crazy storm just came through," he said. "I was at work and it was like the end of the world." My nephew is no wimp, and for him to be rattled got my attention. That and the deep rumbling I heard in the distance.

"A storm can't get from here to there that fast," I decided. But I went back downstairs and returned to the television, a little nervous.

It was Washington, DC, they were talking about after all. And the wind was picking up in a big way. I was a little confused by the suddenness, and I called the backup caregiver who was at Mom's. "Get away from the windows fast," I ordered. "Get two chairs and go into the bathroom until it gets quiet." The storm was moving in quickly. It was ominous. I rounded up the cats and put them in a bathroom. At least I would know where they were if something happened. I clipped on Sasha's leash and sat down on the couch. If it got ugly, we'd get in the bathroom too. To say Sasha was scared was an understatement. She seemed to know something big was coming, and the fifty-pound dog was trying hard to squeeze under the couch and my legs. Now my nephew and my dog had me rattled.

The wind howled and the thunder roared. The lightning was nonstop—bolts and flashes seemed to go on without pause. A large branch crashed onto the roof and bounced over the skylight. Rick was right. It did sort of seem like the end of the world. I called Mom's, and there was no answer. "Good, they are in the bathroom," I thought. The condo was beautiful because of the two oversized sets of sliding glass doors in the living and dining area. Then there were windows in the bedrooms. I worried about broken glass becoming projectiles. Then the power went out. It didn't go out with a flicker or a fizzle. It went down suddenly with a sense of finality. That seemed different.

Sasha and I waited out the rest of the storm in the living room. I called Mom's, and they had ventured out of the bathroom. But her power was off too. When the lightning stopped, I picked up a flashlight and took Sasha out for a walk. It was a hot and steamy summer night. I didn't see any major damage—only branches were down, not trees, and the pavement was littered with debris. "Let's go to bed," I said to Sasha as though she spoke fluent English. There wasn't much left to do.

The next morning, I opened one eye to see if I could see the clock—my indicator of power. None. It was warm too. Wikipedia defines a "derecho" as "a widespread, long-lived, straight-line windstorm that is associated with a fast-moving band of severe thunderstorms." Everyone in DC was learning that definition. It had blown chaos into the city and blown out much of the power. Most traffic lights were out, and businesses—including gas stations—were shut down. I called the caregiver and said it was okay to open the fridge long enough to grab milk for a cereal breakfast.

"Gee, this is weird, isn't it," my friend Sandy said as she walked up with her dog. We decided that the best thing to do would be to go out for breakfast and see how things were looking.

At the time, it seemed like an adventure. That wouldn't last long, though. I drove, and it was obvious we had a problem, passing block after block of dark buildings. But we saw that McDonald's was open as we passed it. "Turn around," Sandy said. "It's open." But most people had already figured out this secret, and the line was out the door. Instead, we drove back to a hotel just a block away from our homes. Surely they would have backup power. They did not, but we feasted on breads, fruits, and other items they tried to get rid of before the heat spoiled them. Somehow they were able to make coffee, which hit the spot.

"I think I have a big problem," I told Sandy over coffee. "I'd better hurry and find a hotel for Mom." It was almost one hundred degrees, and other people would be looking too. The CARE-Assist TB test requirement would knock them out as an option. It was still early, and perhaps I was realizing the gravity of the situation before others. The challenge was cell phones—most calls wouldn't go through. We would learn later that cell towers had been knocked out. So I dropped Sandy off and got out on the road.

Washington drivers are not known for their bad-weather driving skills, and this was evident as people whipped through dark intersections without stopping. Police were at the major ones, but numerous intersections were unprotected. It was treacherous.

I hit the nearby hotels first, with no luck. "My mother has Alzheimer's and is in hospice. It's too hot, and we need help," I would plead.

The front-desk people would look at me apologetically and say, "I'm sorry."

I needed backup, so I called Jennifer on her landline. "Oh, man, I'm so glad you answered," I said. She lived in Annapolis, but they had gotten hit too. "Power is out for Mom and me both. I have to find a hotel." We would spend the next two hours on the hunt, with me driving and her making calls from her landline. Some hotels answered, some not. I had the radio on and would hear them identify hotels that had vacancies, but I couldn't get through on the phone, and by the time I would get there in person, they would be full.

Then my phone rang. "You have reservations at the Crystal City Gateway," Jennifer said quickly. "Get there fast."

"Thank you, thank you!" I exclaimed and hung up.

Traffic was thick as I tried to get back to Mom's. I decided that I would take Mom and the caregiver to the hotel, and I would return to my steamy house and stay with the pets. I stopped at home to walk Sasha and could feel the top floor starting to get hot. Later, the house would bake.

"It might be a good idea to close the blinds and keep the sun out," I said as I walked into Mom's place.

"I like the sunshine," the caregiver said, "and so does your mother."

I didn't take time to explain why this wasn't the best idea, and I closed the blinds myself. Then I shared the plan with Mom and the caregiver, and off we went. "Mom, you get to go to a nice hotel!" I exclaimed. We'd had a family joke for years that Mom wanted to come back in her next life as a hotel reviewer—she loved them.

"Really?" She smiled. "We'll have a great time!"

I explained that I wouldn't be staying, which troubled Mom. "But I'll be there as long as you need me," I promised.

What happened next is the reason I share this particular storm story. The three of us sat down for dinner at the hotel's restaurant. I was bedraggled. It was a beastly hot day, and I was damp with sweat. But it was pleasant sitting next to a big window that overlooked the hotel pool.

"Betty," the caregiver said in her heavy accent, "when Julie leaves, I'm going to throw you in the pool."

"Stop it," I hissed at her. "You cannot say things like that to my mother." She was joking and I could tell, but the cultural divide between them was too great. On what planet was it okay to tell a worried woman with dementia that you were going to throw her into the pool?

The nice thing about Alzheimer's is that people are likely to forget things pretty quickly, which Mom did. But I left with a heavy heart. Many neighbors had left my street, and it was quiet as I pulled into my driveway. Before I climbed into bed—the futon on the first floor, where it wasn't quite as oppressive—I got my brother's gun out and put it on the bathroom counter. The darkness was as oppressive as the heat, and I felt very vulnerable. But with the gun nearby, Chris seemed to be near as well. With the power out, there wasn't much to do those nights except lie awake in the warmth and think. I thought about where we were and where we were going.

It lasted almost a week. Grace returned after the first night in the hotel, and she and Mom spent a second night there. Then I got word that a hotel close by had rooms available, and I grabbed one as fast as I could. The driving between home, work, and the hotel was killing me, and this would be easier. And it was a little suite with a microwave and refrigerator, so I stocked them up with supplies.

Grace was horrified when I told her about the pool comment. "That caregiver was different before," Grace said. "She used to be good, but I saw a change." So had I.

Deepening Suspicion
When we finally made it home at the end of the week, Grace and I were sitting in the condo with the air conditioner blasting when she said, "CARE-Home said they will fire me if I talk to you about the caregivers. They said you only complain because I tell you there is something wrong. And they said you cannot hire me if they fire me, or they will come after me."

"Grace," I said sternly, "I am the one who will fire you if you put my mother in danger by not telling me when there is a problem. You cannot work for me if you don't promise to tell me if there is a problem. I will not throw you under the bus."

She looked at me quizzically after the bus part. "I will not give you up," I explained. Besides, Grace wasn't the reason I was complaining. I could tell the quality of the back-up caregivers in ten minutes, just like Grace, but I also had the camera.

"Ju-lee, please be careful," she said. Now I was on alert. This was the third time, and there was no confusion.

"Is there something more I should know?" I asked. Grace looked away, but something didn't feel right.

We had been through more chaos, but I still felt like Mom was in the right place. After all, CARE-Assist could lose power too. The only difference was they were on a high-priority list for restoration. We weren't.

We didn't have long to recover from the storm before the next disaster struck. I had just gotten to work one day when my phone rang.

"Lots of water in your Mom's bathroom," Grace said hurriedly.

"Turn off the toilet!" I instructed, lacking a better suggestion.

Grace's tone was urgent when she got back to the phone. "More water—it can't be the toilet."

"Run to the management office! Please move fast," I responded.

There wasn't much I could do to help from work, so I waited for an update. Moments later the management office called. "A pipe burst, and we need to rip out drywall to get to it," they said. "It's bad. Do we have your permission?"

"Yes, please move fast," I said flatly. Really? How much damage had occurred during the time it took to make that call? I'd find out later that the water had done a lot of damage, taking out large chunks of the bathroom, the closet, and the carpet before they could get it shut off. Still, I hadn't trained well enough, I decided. Grace should have just run for the management office. What if I hadn't answered the phone? Caregivers need to know what to do in emergencies.

>>> Care Point 21 <<<
Think of as many types of emergencies as you can—and train for them.

That evening, as I surveyed the damage—which was worse than I was expecting—I decided that when times are tough, it just seems like everything is going wrong. The mishaps are magnified. In reality, I think they are always there. On good days, you just don't notice them as much. I always tried to look for the brighter side, and now I reminded myself that the management staff hadn't waited for insurance appraisers. They had brought in huge fans and dehumidifiers to get ahead of the mold risk. That was a bright side—more strangers looking out for us.

Mom was steadily getting worse, but we continued to get out for church and meals. Hospice was coming regularly, but it was hard to say where we really were in this cycle of Alzheimer's. Mom was loved by everyone she knew. She had rock-star status at several local restaurants, and groups of employees would frequently greet her as her entourage came in (some combination of Cindy, Pat, Grace, and me). They would stop and talk—they truly cared about her and me. Some of my friendships had taken a beating during these years and fizzled. But I was very aware of the new people who had come into my life as a result—friends and caring people who jumped into the gap unexpectedly.

For a long time, Grace joined us for church. But then she suddenly stopped. So I would pick Mom up for church, lunch, and some fun activity and bring her back as late in the day as possible.

It never failed: Mom and I would get settled at church, and I would need to go to the ladies' room. For a long time, I could say to Mom, "You sit here, and I'll be right back." And it was fine. But as time went on, that was riskier. I'd plan ahead, of course, but sometimes it couldn't be helped. One Sunday, I made the usual statement to her and walked to the door of the sanctuary not too far away. Luckily I looked back, because Mom had gotten out of her wheelchair and was standing. "Oops!" I said audibly and ran back to her. We sat back down, and a few minutes later, a woman tapped me on the shoulder. She had been in the balcony behind us and had seen me run.

"I'll sit with your mom while you go to the ladies' room," she said.

These little encounters meant so much to me—small, kind things that people did. On a different Sunday, Mom refused to sit down after we had stood up (carefully and awkwardly) to sing. Mom always wanted to stand when everyone else did. Sometimes I would tell a fib, saying that my leg was hurting, and ask her if she'd stay seated with me. She would look irritated but would say *okay*. But this time I just couldn't get her to sit. I could feel my face flushing as I tried and tried and we blocked the people behind us. I gave up and we started to walk, with Mom on my arm and me pulling the chair behind me.

"Don't leave!" I heard a woman's voice say. "Just let her stand—we'll be fine." Everyone around her nodded in agreement.

"Thanks," I responded, and we returned to where we had been. I really needed to be there that day, and their kindness meant a lot. Ironically, Mom sat back down.

The weekend of the storm, I had been scheduled to fly to Boston to visit with Erica. She was working there for the summer. She was in love with the city and wanted me to come. I wanted to share it with her and was determined to go. But I had postponed it in the aftermath of the storm. We picked August 17 to try again.

CHAPTER 17

Losing Grace

t all happened on such a perfect day. That's what I still can't figure out. It was August 5, 2012. Mom and I had been to church, and we picked Grace up afterward for lunch. Pat and Hailey joined us, and our table was the source of laughter and talking. Mom wasn't too much a part of the conversation by this time, but I would do the talking for her by saying things like, "Mom, you remember that...remember when I sent..."

Mom would say, "Oh yes, I remember," as though she really did. It let her feel a part of things.

The day was particularly happy—it was a rare day where I wasn't feeling overwhelmed, and we lingered over coffee. Pat headed home, leaving Hailey to spend the afternoon with me. Hailey is one of the many kids in my life. What's that saying— "Always a bridesmaid, never a bride"? Well, with me, it's "Always a godmother, never a mother." And that has turned out to be okay. Hailey had a special relationship with Mom. She has a sweet and thoughtful heart and no fear. And on this day, she wanted to help me with chores at the house. But first, Hailey, Grace, Mom, and I strolled around the mall, before ending up at a toy store.

"Let's buy Grandbet a new doll," Hailey said.

"Great idea, let's do," I agreed.

Mom had another doll that she loved. Two wouldn't hurt. Hailey picked out one of the ones you fill with water to make soft and cuddly. "Look, Julie," she said, "Grandbet reached for this one. This must be the one she wants."

We headed for home. Hailey and I dropped Mom and Grace off, and I said I'd be back soon. "Ju-lee, please print big pictures for me," Grace requested as we left. Her son-in-law had sent me beautiful photos of Grace's granddaughters, and I had printed small ones for her. But she liked big, full-page photos. I had bought large frames for her, and she was reminding me she needed the pictures to match. By this time, I even had an e-mail relationship with Grace's son-in-law, who lived in Nigeria. He was a trainer, and I had bought him a membership in my training organization as a gift. We had tried in vain to get him to the United States for our annual conference, but he wasn't able to get a visa. We had agreed to redouble our efforts the following year. Our families had become linked in more ways than one.

At my house, Hailey vacuumed and played with Sasha as I paid a few bills. But as we got ready to go, a storm swept in. We sat and talked awhile to let it pass. It probably delayed us fifteen minutes.

Hailey and I were talking as we walked. She's a great kid and probably as talkative as I am. Which is to say, talkative. At first our chatting blocked out the yelling. But as we approached Mom's place, I became aware of it, and I froze. The yelling was violent—not like someone was snapping at someone else, saying, "Don't do that." It was screaming without taking a breath. It was rage. And it was Grace. Now we were one unit away—the next door would be Mom's—and I had no doubt.

"Who's yelling?" Hailey asked. I was stunned and didn't answer as I quietly and quickly got my key out. "Should I knock?" she asked.

I pushed her back as I hissed, "No!" I had gotten good at silently getting my key in the lock and walking in unannounced. I had done it many times to keep the element of surprise on my side, especially with the backup caregivers, but even with Grace.

The look on Mom's face is etched in my memory—hollow, sad, and defeated. She was sitting on the edge of her "geri chair," as it was called—a chair for people with mobility issues. Grace was standing nearby.

"What is going on here?" I heard my voice boom.

Hailey had walked in on my heels, and the awful look on Mom's face melted into a big smile as she saw her young friend. I said it again, in shock, "*What* is going on here?"

"Walk, walk, walk...I was afraid she was going to fall, walk, walk, walk," Grace said. Her words were tumbling out, and she kept repeating them. "She was like this," Grace wept, and she tried to demonstrate, knocking breakables off the shelves and raising her voice to a shout again.

"Stop it, Grace!" I ordered in a loud voice. My brain could not comprehend what was happening. No voices were ever raised at my mom's. Grace was normally calm, slow moving, and methodical. A mountain of a woman, both literally and figuratively. "Hailey," I said, "why don't you and Grandbet stay here in the living room? I need to talk to Grace in the bedroom."

We stepped into Grace's room and closed the door. "Just stop it. Stop it!" I said. "Take a deep breath and calm down. Has this ever happened before?" I implored. Grace was silent. "Grace, have you ever yelled at my mother before?"

I never got an answer. She went into her "walk, walk, walk" rant again. "Stop it, Grace!" I ordered again. "You can never, ever, ever raise your voice to my mother. How could you? How could you do this?" I was still having trouble comprehending what had happened. My mind was scrambling to put the pieces together. And it couldn't.

Grace didn't say much once she calmed down, only that she'd gotten worried and had panicked. Eventually we joined Mom and Hailey. Mom was holding one of the dolls, and she looked more like herself. Hailey was looking at me quizzically and kept talking to Mom.

We stayed awhile, and calm returned. But it was an uneasy calm. "Hailey, I'd better take you home," I said, and we made the short drive to Pat's.

"Grandma, something happened," she said to Pat as I collapsed on the couch.

Pat froze. "What happened?"

I explained the afternoon's events. Hailey kept repeating, "Why would Grace yell at Grandbet?"

"I don't know," I said. "I don't know. I have to get to the camera." I stood up to leave. "I'll call Phil and Barbara. I need them." Later I drove back to Mom's, and all was quiet. Mom was asleep. Grace and I didn't talk about what had happened. But she was different. It was an eerie calm.

Standing in my living room, with both Phil and Barbara's cells going to voice mail, I had a growing sense of dread. What had happened? I played Grace's voice over and over again in my head.

There was no answer and no returned phone calls from Barbara and Phil. They must be on vacation, I decided. They wouldn't ignore my repeated calls if they were getting them. They would have known that near-simultaneous calls to both of them would have signaled trouble.

I lay in bed, worried and unable to sleep. I had to get to the camera. "I shouldn't have left them there," I thought. I waited until six the next morning to call Pat. "Phil and Barbara must be out of town," I told her. "You have to go to Mom's and borrow the clock radio."

"Got it. I'll go over as soon as Hailey gets here," she responded.

Next I called Tony. "I need to look at our camera, so I'll be late," I said. "I think it should be fine, and I'll be in soon."

Despite my worry, I still couldn't imagine seeing something terrible. As I pored through the camera card, Pat and Hailey talked worriedly. "Why would Grace yell at Grandbet?" Hailey asked. "I don't understand."

It's tedious to navigate around the camera card, but I located the hour before Hailey and I had walked in. It started with Grace putting Mom in her chair and Mom getting up. As I watched, I could see Grace starting to get more forceful with Mom—pushing her repeatedly instead of gently guiding her, and Mom getting up repeatedly. Then Mom's face started to show pain—and anger. There was no sound, but you could see her mouth the word "Ow!" and she held her arm where it hurt and glared angrily at Grace. The dance continued. Grace pushed her down, and Mom got back up.

Perhaps it was the repetition. Perhaps Grace had gotten bad news—in the video she was walking with what appeared to be a phone in her hand. Perhaps it was the lack of training, which was evident with hindsight. But Grace snapped. We watched in horror as Mom got out of her chair, began walking toward the door (probably to try and leave out of anger), and started to have one of her episodes like I had witnessed in the past—"the look," only this time I wasn't there to catch her. She started to crumple. Grace rushed over, but instead of gently catching her as we typically would, Grace grabbed her and pushed her toward the chair. Mom was fragile and slow moving, and everyone who knew her knew that her feet wouldn't handle a push. Down she went—and Grace, tripping, went down on top of her. I can't guess weight very well, but I suspect Grace was well over twice my size. She dwarfed my 130-pound frame and Mom's now-120-pound frame. In anger, Grace used Mom's back to get up. She actually put her full weight on Mom twice as she rose to her feet. And then you saw the screaming—sheer and uncontrolled anger. It struck me as evil, what I saw in her face—inches away from Mom's ear. Mom was prone, and Grace jerked her to a sitting position. Mom fell back down, and Grace did it again. Who knows what Mom said to this angry, out-of-control woman who was treating her this way in her own home, but it caused Grace to slap her. Grace stepped over her, still screaming, and Mom slapped her on the leg. Grace probably didn't even feel it, but even as I watched in horror, I was happy she'd tried to hit Grace, however feebly.

I felt sick. But it got worse. Grace ended up—all while screaming uncontrollably—pulling Mom by the ankles toward her chair, roughly picking Mom up by her chest, and dropping her into her chair, and then hitting her again in the arm.

"Oh God, oh God..." was all I could muster. I had jumped to my feet and knocked the chair backward.

"Julie, sit down," Pat said firmly. "You have to get this right."

I knew she was right. Do you know that phrase "It felt like a kick in the stomach"? Well, that's real. There was a piercing pain in my right side, and it hurt terribly to stand. Oddly, all I could think of was my brother. "Why aren't you here? I need you," I thought.

But even in this grim situation, I had time to think about how I was probably wrong about that. I think my brother could have killed Grace. Or at least hurt her. He was fiercely protective of his family, I knew. He had much more of a temper than I. And the man always carried a gun. I could have multiple problems on my hands if Chris were here.

We watched the video several more times, studying it and noticing more horror and more detail each time. "How could Grace do this?" Hailey implored over and over again.

"I don't know," I kept repeating.

Detective Allen was the one to answer the phone when I called their number—no nine one one this time, as I knew the detectives who'd handled the thefts would remember me. I don't think I was making sense, but it was enough. "Hold on," he said. "This is out of our area. Sit near your phone, and I'm going to have someone call you back."

I hung up, turned to Pat, and said, "Get to Mom's."

Hailey said, "I'm scared. What if she does something to us?"

"She won't," I assured her. "Just go over and hang out with her and Mom like you've done before. Play with dolls. Do whatever."

Off they went to keep my mother safe, and I sat at the kitchen table watching the phone and waiting for it to ring. "That clock is so loud," I thought. "Does it have to tick that way?" Silence is truly deafening. I called Tony and said in a rushed voice that didn't sound quite right in my ears, "I found something on the video. My mom was assaulted. I'm waiting for the police."

"Oh God," he said.

It wasn't long before Detective Mullins arrived. We sat at my kitchen table, watching and rewatching the video. We slowed it and watched every detail. "Look at Grace's face," I said tearfully. "Look at the anger. Look at my Mom's face!" Mom was angry too, but she was no match for Grace. She looked defeated.

"Ms. Nielsen, I don't want you to think because of what I'm about to say that we will in any way minimize what happened," Detective Mullins said. "But it's misdemeanor assault on an incapacitated adult. It's not a felony because your mom wasn't seriously injured."

Misdemeanor? That sounded so minor. The CARE-Assist thefts had been misdemeanors. This was different. This wasn't about money. It wasn't about pilfering twenty-dollar bills out of a wallet. It was about violence and physical assault.

"Let's go," the detective said. "I'll follow you over. Get everyone out of the unit except Grace. I want to talk to her with as little notice as possible."

"Sorry, you can't park there," the security manager said as we walked in, leaving both our cars sitting in front.

"He's on official business, Jill," I said. Jill was an ally and fierce protector of my mom. In her role as security manager at the Renaissance, she had helped us many times.

The detective pulled out his badge, and Jill looked stricken. She turned to me, saying in a panicked voice, "What's wrong?"

"I'll talk to you later," I said quietly.

The detective was behind me as I walked into Mom's. Pat looked grim as she stood up. Hailey had been sitting with Mom. Ruth was there too—the fact that it was Monday was lost on me in the turmoil. I had forgotten that she'd be coming, as she usually did on Mondays, and she was oblivious to what was happening. Mom was already sitting in her wheelchair. "Everyone," I announced, "we need to all go downstairs." I turned to Grace, who was standing in the dining room, and said, "Grace, this is Detective Mullins with the Fairfax County police. He'd like to talk with you."

Pat was rushing to get everyone out. "Okay," was all Grace said. She didn't look to me to be overly concerned.

I was numb. We walked silently down the long hall to the elevators, with Hailey pushing Mom in the chair. "What is going on?" Ruth said incredulously.

"Let's get to the lobby. I'll let Pat explain while I make a phone call."

"Am I glad I moved Mom from CARE-Assist?" I thought. For the first time, I wavered on my answer. But when I look back on it all, the most important thing I learned was that no option was perfect. Assisted-living facilities, or in-home assisted living—both could have serious if not fatal flaws. Both had advantages and disadvantages, risks, and rewards. Both require vigilance and aggressive involvement by family members.

Two Reactions, Worlds Apart

"Please get the most senior person available on the phone right away," I said to the receptionist at CARE-Home. Lynn, the manager of the caregivers, was on the phone fast. Clearly my request had been shared with her by the time she got on the phone.

"There are three things you need to know," I started. "First, someone senior needs to get to Mom's immediately. Second, you need to find a new caregiver immediately. And third, you need to know that a Fairfax County police detective is interviewing Grace about an assault on my mother." In the craziness that was unfolding, that was my life, I wasn't even thinking about where the next caregiver should come from. I just knew I needed help.

"Who called the police?" was Lynn's angry answer.

I was stunned and silent for a second. Somehow I remained calm. "I called the police. There has been an assault on my mom."

"How could you not call us first?" she implored.

"Just come," I said.

"Who called the police? *Who called the police?*" I was thinking wildly. These nice but naïve women wanted to be the first to investigate? I don't think so. I never questioned that call, and her response sounded silly as I mulled it over repeatedly.

Lynn was on a tear when she came through the front door of the Renaissance. "What is going on?" she said angrily.

"I walked in on yelling yesterday," I said calmly. I had knowledge on my side, and she was walking in blind.

"Yelling? Yelling?" she almost shouted. "This is about yelling?"

"No, I saw the whole thing." It was probably seconds that ticked by, but it seemed like minutes.

"You have a camera," she said in a resigned voice.

"We have a camera," I said. I'm not sure which was worse—her anger at me calling the police or her anger over the camera.

"How could you not trust us?" she started back in.

"Lynn, this is not about trust. It's about me protecting my mother, which I just did—unfortunately, after the fact." I stopped her from heading for the elevator. "The detective said he doesn't want anyone coming up until he comes down for us."

I was stunned by her response. Neither on the phone nor here in person did she ask how my mother was. Her concern was clearly elsewhere—I couldn't tell where. I remembered the CARE-Assist manager's words after I had called about the thief: "Thank you for doing exactly what you did, exactly how you did it, exactly when you did it. Thank you for protecting everyone in the building, as well as CARE-Assist. We'll be there with you." The contrast was vividly clear.

It would be the last I saw of any CARE-Home employee for a long time. The rug had been pulled out from under us.

That day was the end of my innocence and blind trust. Grace stole my ability to trust that day, and I don't know if I'll ever fully get it back.

Overwhelming Doubt

The horror of it all began to wash over me. Had Grace been abusing my mother all along? Or had she simply snapped? I thought back to unexplained bruises that had appeared periodically over the more than three years that Grace was with us. And bloody bed linens that Grace said were from bloody noses. Fragile people fall. And ill people get nosebleeds. But was it a fall, or was it Grace? Were they nosebleeds or something worse? I thought back to the shortage of breaks Grace had taken. "This is what they do, Julie," I had been told by CARE-Home when I asked them about it. I thought too about the fact that we had let Grace into our family, albeit with a camera nearby. I had let her cross the line from employee to family member. And that was a mistake.

>>> **Care Point 22** <<<
Consider rotating caregivers so that one person isn't stuck with a trying client for too long.

"Julie, don't do this!" Grace was crying. "I love your mother. I love you." She had me by the arms.

As I'd entered Mom's unit, Detective Mullins said, "Grace, stay away from Julie. Do not touch her." But she had grabbed me immediately. She was strong, and I felt fear briefly as I contemplated what she had done to Mom. I couldn't get away. "Let go of her," the detective was ordering.

"Please don't do this," Grace kept crying.

"Elbow surgery, right arm," I said to the detective, hoping that I wasn't about to have my tendon torn again. But Grace heard and let go.

"Ju-lee, I didn't push your mom," she said through tears. "I didn't push your mom."

"This isn't about pushing," I said. "I saw the whole thing, Grace." I wanted to believe her, but the video couldn't lie, as Grace was. And she was very believable. That was disturbing. The detective had told her there was a camera and had cautioned me about providing too many details. "I saw the whole thing," I kept repeating. The video, and the violence of it, were fresh in my brain. I could see Grace's face, inches from Mom's, screaming violently. And I could hear Lynn's voice: "You called the police?"

Grace realized it was happening. I wasn't changing my mind. She was leaving. She was supposed to pack just a few necessities and get out, allowing CARE-Home to get her fully moved out later. But she ended up packing everything. That was probably better. I needed to close this chapter, and although I didn't know it then, CARE-Home would be disappearing too. Skillfully, and even artfully, CARE-Home called another caregiving company for backup. The CEO and a manager showed up quickly. I recognized the company name—CARE-Home had called them once when they were out of backup caregivers. Oddly, at the time I had been impressed with them and wondered if I should switch. They were current, customer focused, and used technology well. They were involved. The CEO had called me even back then, for that one brief backup, and said to call him if I ever needed anything. "No," I had thought, "better stay with who I know, no matter how frumpy and nontechnical." Ironically, years later they would purchase CARE-Home.

I don't remember calling hospice, but I must have. They showed up to check Mom over. Although she didn't show any signs of broken bones, her mental state had changed. That would become clearer over the next two weeks. Late in the day, I left a message for my doctor to call me—the one who'd advised me not to look for monsters. It didn't take long—he could tell something was wrong.

"You have to look for monsters," I said when I answered the phone. "Monsters can be beautiful, and you might miss them." I explained my two-day odyssey, and we agreed as we hung up: "You have to look for monsters." Grace and our thief, our two criminals, were beautiful. Monsters don't wear signs identifying themselves.

Grace wasn't arrested that day. The police had me go back through the camera cards to determine if I had unknowingly captured other examples of abuse. It was tedious and took several days. There were a few concerning clips leading up to the incident, but nothing that rose to the felony level. An arrest warrant was issued shortly after.

The Aftermath

This brings me back to the training plan. Earlier I talked about basic household maintenance and then crisis planning. But perhaps the most important part of the plan is what to do when you can't take it anymore. And this was a huge gap. I didn't know how to plan for this. It was now one of those "hindsight is twenty-twenty" moments, and it did not appear that CARE-Home knew to plan for it either. Grace had had several options that day. She could have called me, and I could have been there in five minutes; after all, she knew I was at home. She could have called her company and asked for a break. She could have even locked Mom in the condo and gone for a walk—not ideal, but better than her ultimate choice. Instead she lost all control and took it out on Mom.

Caregiver Training Plan

If you have a loved one in an assisted-living facility, especially a corporate one such as I used, you can most likely count on quality training in basic caregiving. But you should inquire as to their crisis plan. How do they get residents out if the building is damaged? Where would they go in the case of a regional crisis?

In-home caregiving is another story, whether you have a caregiving company or you hire someone privately. Create a training notebook (hard copy, since caregivers are unlikely to have computers with them). Regardless of how long the person works for your family, drill on the plan on a set schedule.

The components of your plan should include the following:

1. Basic household maintenance, with contact information in your absence
2. Food safety according to your standards
3. DNR: use if a Do Not Resuscitate order is in place. What is it, when is it used, and why is it important?
4. Medical crisis handling—who gets called first, and what's the backup?
5. Structural crisis handling—what should they do in case of fire, earthquake, or other crises?
6. Options when you run out of patience—what do you do when you can't take it anymore?

Two things changed right away. First, ADT (the well-known security company) would come through in a big way. They were at Mom's the next day, and we figured out how to wire the condo for visible cameras. We would end up with one big camera—the kind in a bubble, frequently seen in buildings—that was always taping in the living room, storing sixty days at a time in case I needed it. There was a smaller camera in the kitchen and another one in the bedroom, with the ability to see the bathroom as well. I wasn't concerned about Mom's privacy at this point. I was focused on her safety. My ability to trust was demolished. All three cameras had infrared capability and could see in the dark. In the darkness, the picture turned to black and white but remained crystal clear. In the light, the picture was in color and vivid. But the biggest benefit was that I (or any friend, if I wanted to share access) could watch Mom via computer, iPhone, or iPad at any time.

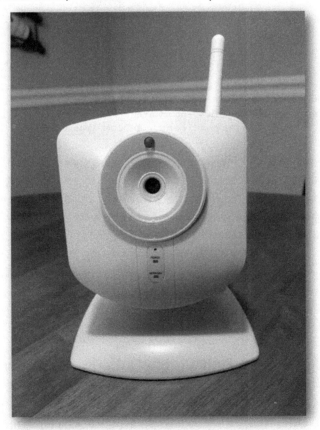

One of the cameras in use in the condo after the assault

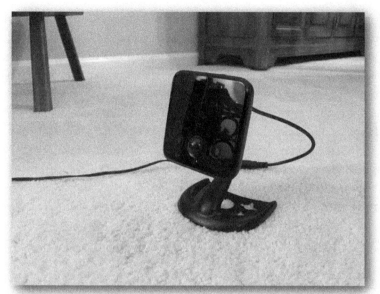

Another type of camera in use in the condo; this one uses infrared technology that allows the camera to see in the dark. There was a traditional "bubble camera" on the wall, catching and saving all activity in the main part of the condo. All of them could be accessed by smartphone or tablet.

Ironically, when sharing my experience with friends and acquaintances who had parents already caught in the headlights of Alzheimer's, I would tell them to get a nanny cam. This was before the assault. After the assault, I would say, "Call ADT and get the real thing. The nanny cam is hard to use because you need access to it when no one is around." Plus, I had learned that the threat of someone watching provided some safety. But above all, you can't backup. You can't get to know someone and then say, "By the way, I want to install cameras." You need to do it before the caregiver walks in the door, and be public about it. Make no mistake: when you have others caring for physically or mentally incapacitated people, cameras are a requirement—whichever care route you go.

Technology Tool #4: Fully Visible Cameras (with or without Monitoring)

Visible cameras require more of an investment than a nanny cam, but they can now be quite reasonably priced. And they keep everyone safe, not just your loved one. What happened is never in question. If they are already installed when a caregiver first arrives, then it's a done deal from day one. There is no secrecy and no help required. You can watch your loved one from a smartphone or tablet at any time. You can choose to have cameras capture and keep footage in case something happens while you're not watching.

Much later, Sue would tell me over lunch one day that she had hired elder consultants to oversee her mom's care when she moved out of CARE-Assist—people totally separate from the caregiving company. In hindsight, that was a missing piece of the puzzle my mother and I lived in. One company was providing care, saying they were providing training and serving as eyes and ears. It was like a fox keeping an eye on the henhouse. No outsider was observing and looking for trouble, and as a business, there was an incentive to just make things go smoothly. There was a lot of money changing hands and a big incentive to keep it flowing. In the end, the likelihood of trouble would have been noticeable to an outsider.

"They had me fire the caregiver I liked best," Sue said that day.

"What did they see?" I asked.

"They could see that, although the caregiver seemed to love my mom, she couldn't handle the stress and frustration created by someone with repetitive behavior driven by dementia. They could see a problem coming. And they said she had to go." There was no attachment and no concern for the business aspect. The focus had been on the most important person—Sue's mom.

>>> Care Point 23 <<<
Who is your care advisor looking out for—your parent or the company?

Care Concept #11: Clarify and Separate Caregiving Roles

If you choose to go the in-home caregiving route, there are two types of organizations you need to be aware of: the caregiving agencies and caregiving advisors.

You need a caregiving agency if you want to employ a company to provide caregiving in your home, a loved one's home, or some other location.

You need a caregiving advisor regardless. These advisors have backgrounds in geriatric fields and have seen much more than you have. They know more than you do—about options, finances, and logistics.

Don't use one company for both services. The advisor should put you or your loved one first and have no ties to the business of caregiving. Keep the lines—and the roles—clear.

Mom was dying. She was dying before the attack, but this was different. She was frailer and less mentally capable afterward. We all saw it. I tried to put on a happy face and pretend that everything was okay. But I knew it wasn't. The new company had found a good caregiver named Maria. She seemed wonderful, but I kept her at arm's length. I couldn't let my guard down again. I was at Mom's a lot, and Maria and I would talk every time. She was in this for the long haul, I could tell.

"Why do you have the cameras?" she asked one night when we sat with Mom at the dining room table. I gave her a brief summary. "I'll never mistreat your mother," she said, locking eyes with me. Still, my guard had to stay up.

I decided to keep my date with Erica in Boston. I wouldn't be gone long. I had a sense of foreboding and that our time would be important. August 17 rolled around. Our volunteer with hospice, whom I adored, came for a visit while I was there. "Your mom is different," she said. "Something happened in the attack."

"I think so too," I said, "but the nurse said nothing was visibly wrong." But I wasn't the only one seeing it, and I called Dr. Lessin's office. His nurse updated him.

"I just faxed you an order for an MRI," she said when she called me back.

"Here goes Boston and my break," I thought. I hated to disappoint Erica again. And I needed my own break. I shared my sad story with the MRI scheduler on the other end of the phone line after she said there would be a delay.

"Can you come now?" she said.

"We're on our way!" Maria and I got Mom in the car and up the street to the MRI office, where they worked us in between appointments.

"In light of what's going on, the radiologist went ahead and looked at the results," the nurse said. "No sign of a major head injury." I had told her a lot of my story. "Get to the airport," she said with a smile. "I think you'll need it." Mom looked content but far away in her wheelchair. We left for home, and within an hour, I was in a taxi headed for the airport and a welcome break.

Boston was a breath of fresh air. Everyone should hang out with a twenty-one-year-old. We shopped, got massages, went to movies, and did what I had looked forward to for years: as a teen, Erica had been staying with me on one of her weekend trips when she said, "I'm looking forward to being twenty-one and having a glass of wine with you before a nice meal." It had stayed with me. In Boston, we would have that meal and a grown-up niece and Aunt Julie talking as friends.

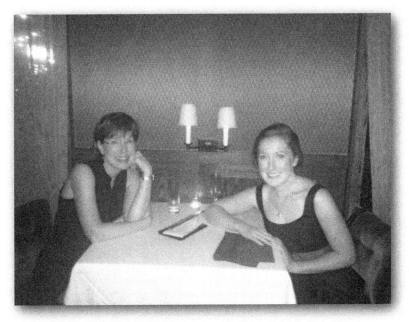

Erica and me at our grown-up dinner, after a day of fun in Boston

But I was haunted. What happened was always in the back of my mind. One thing in particular bothered me: the blood on the bedspread. Grace kept saying Mom was having bloody noses. I'd had no reason to doubt her—until now.

CHAPTER 18

Losing My Best Friend

Flying back into DC that Sunday afternoon, my sense of foreboding was back. Things weren't right, and I knew it. Mom was vacant and unaware. I knew I was losing her.

"Come quickly, Julie," Maria said the following Friday night. "Something happened to your mom."

I rushed over. She was in bed but even more listless. I couldn't get her up and couldn't get a response. The camera came in handy. I was able to look at history on my phone and see what had happened. Maria was trying to get Mom into bed, and Mom seemed to go rigid. There was clearly some sort of an event. I didn't need hospice to tell me what was happening, although I called and asked them to come. I knew.

People came and went. I spent more time there but kept working too. We had no idea how long it would be. But that following week, after a glimpse of improvement where the hospice volunteer was able to get Mom out of bed and into a chair, we rolled downhill. "Maria will need to leave," the company's manager was telling me. Another change in a sea of changes. We were about to add major narcotic drugs for Mom, and nurses (LPNs) would be required to dispense them. The first night we used them, I did it myself, sleeping for a few hours in between. I decided I needed sleep, and they were right about needing nurses. Maria was a lovely woman, and it was hard for her to leave. My mom had that kind of power. Even at the end, her warmth, gentleness, and sweetness were clear. Even though I had kept my guard up, I cried as we said goodbye. It wasn't the last time I would see her.

Mom was almost asleep, but not quite. I would talk and talk to her, and so would the caregivers and the hospice visitors. My focus was Mom, but the realization that I was about to be a forty-eight-year-old orphan was creeping into my mind. "I can't believe I got here," I would think. "How could I lose Dad, Chris, and Mom—all by forty-eight?" I had lots of time to think. And I could make myself laugh. I recalled how Chris and I had joked. "When we get old," I would quip, "I'll clip the hair in your ears if you'll pull the whiskers on my chin." Mom's ability to see her whiskers had declined early, and now I hoped I wouldn't have a beard. I had a wealth of stories running through my mind. Laughter was embedded in the Nielsen family, and I treasured my mental library of funny stories and images.

Rick and Erica drove up on August 31, Friday. "We'll have the weekend," I thought. I secretly hoped it would happen while they were here. The idea of being alone when Mom died seemed unimaginable. Ruth came over Saturday, and we pored through the photo albums, laughing as we went. The kids were seeing the family history in unusual detail. Their father was on every page, and we seemed to celebrate family, not just my mom. The weekend was good, and we did what we knew Mom would want— we went to dinner and a movie Saturday night.

"I will know," the caregiver said. "It's not time. Go do something with your niece and nephew."

Sitting there in the movie theater, I felt like an observer to my own life, going through the motions. I decided then what I would do the next day. I'd heard stories of people hanging on and not dying until loved ones arrived. Or hanging on until loved ones said, "It's okay." Was Mom hanging on for me? Could she see through the fog of Alzheimer's? I wondered. I decided to tell her the next day everything she needed to know—that I would be okay.

Sunday morning came fast, and I knew the kids would need to leave. I sat down with pen, paper, and coffee in the early-morning silence and began to make my list. It was a list of everything I was and would be because of her. Handwritten on two small pieces of paper. As I finished, the kids got up. The next day was Labor Day, and there was the first day of school to prepare for. Their dad would have been here with me, but I didn't feel like it was their time to witness this. I fought back tears as I waved good-bye and thought of all the times I had wondered if it would be the last time they would see Mom. This time I knew it was.

Once again, I took my laptop and speakers over to Mom's. We would attend church online, as we had that day in the hospital. The caregiver, Erika, attended with us. Afterward, I looked over at Erika, and she had tears in her eyes. "What's wrong?" I asked. She told me that her mom had been trying to get her to go back to church. Her family had been devastated by the economy, and life was upside down.

"I feel like I am here for a reason," she said. "There is something about your family." I knew she was right.

Hospice and caregivers came and went. Pat and Hailey came and stayed. In the midafternoon, I got the list out and read it to Mom. It was a struggle. It's hard to say "I'm okay" through tears and sound like you are really okay. I wasn't, but in my heart, I knew I would be. And I was ready too.

"Please call me if anything changes," Hailey pleaded as they left, late.

"I'll call your grandma, and we'll see what time it is."

"Call me," Pat said with a hug as they left. "I will come." She had been through this with her dad, and it meant so much that she could still show up here with me and see it again.

Mom's death appeared to be imminent. There was a change in caregivers around eight o'clock, but instead of leaving, Erika sat on one side of me and the fresh caregiver sat on the other. I leaned on the bed, keeping Mom's hand in mine and talking to her. Every breath seemed like it might be her last. Finally, Erika got up to leave. "I'll talk to you tomorrow," she said and left, leaving the two of us to our vigil.

And then it happened, or so we thought—the last breath. The caregiver and I studied Mom for what seemed like eternity. She looked at her watch and noted the time of death. "That's it?" I thought. I stared at Mom and looked painstakingly for any sign of life. I was numb. And then she gasped and started breathing again. We actually laughed. "My mom doesn't give up easily," I said. And so began our final vigil.

We sat in chairs on each side of the bed. I dozed off and on, waking frequently to watch Mom—stuck somewhere between sleep and death. Weeks later, I would say to my friend Steve at work, "Why didn't you tell me what death was like?" His father had died the year before, with Steve at his side.

He said with tears in his eyes, "I couldn't talk about it, and I still can't." We would both brush away tears and talk about something inane. Death was awful. I know where I'm headed when I die. But it's the act of dying that is awful. I can't talk about it now either.

Erika, the caregiver, called in the morning. I told her Mom was still with us. "I can't believe it didn't happen," she said quietly. "Are you okay?"

"Yes," I said numbly. But I wasn't okay. It was awful. I'd heard people say it was an honor to be with someone when they died. I couldn't call it that. Death is the subject of many books—but not mine. I just have to tell a story to help others.

"Maybe something else is supposed to happen before she goes," Erika said as she hung up. The caregiver and I assumed our positions, and on the vigil went.

"I need to figure out my career," the caregiver said, somewhat out of the blue. It seemed like a funny thing to comment on when someone was lying in bed dying. But comments like that always draw my attention. I am passionate about helping people obtain jobs, keep jobs, and develop their careers.

"Maybe I can help," I said and told her what I did for a living. And we started to talk, with my eyes trained on Mom. Quietly, Mom's breathing stopped. We both stared, again for what seemed like an eternity. But this time there was no gasp—no return. The caregiver got out her watch. It was the time of death. I wondered if Mom had let go when she heard me helping the caregiver. As in, "my work is done, and my daughter can help others now." My best friend was gone. It was Labor Day morning, 2012.

CHAPTER 19

Saying Good-Bye

had been to Mom's funeral many times in my mind. I had known for years I would do the eulogy. "No way," said several friends, "you'll never make it through." After all, I cry at Hallmark commercials and melt in sad movies. I knew they were wrong, but I arranged for Tony to serve as backup just in case. "Don't worry if I cry," I told him. "Just worry if I lose control and can't get it back."

The planning with the church seemed to flow easily—everything fell into place. As planned, Dale, the pastor from my church, conducted the service.

It felt like I was watching someone else walk to the stage. I had carefully planned the funeral with a kind man from the church. And now it was my time to honor Mom, to capture her life in about fifteen minutes. My life over the last eight years had frequently horrified people. How would I honor my mother and show them that, as horrible as things sometimes got, I was still standing?

What I Said: The Eulogy for Betty Nielsen

Several of you said there is no way I can do this, and we're about to find out. If I can't do it, then my boss, Tony, is going to finish for me. And if he can't do it, then I guess we'll call me done, and I'll e-mail it to everyone.

I started writing this eulogy over a year ago. But like many things in the last few years, it didn't get done. So three nights ago, I sat down to complete it.

The name was originally "What I Will Say." But as I sat there Friday night, I changed it to "What I Said." The previous Sunday I made a list of the things I am and will be because of Mom. Those things became the basis of what I want to share today.

Some of you knew my mom well, and others not at all. I can't paint a picture of her life in the few minutes I have here today. But I thought about what happened when my dad died twenty-one years ago. My friends and I were twenty-seven, and no one ever thought we would lose a parent. And because of Dad's death, several people reconciled with their parents. I remember thinking how pleased he would have been by this.

Something similar happened when my brother, Chris, died. Siblings weren't supposed to die at our age. The preciousness and unpredictability of life rocked my circle of friends. I am an unfortunate trailblazer.

My dad was laid to rest amid the sound of bullets, buried with honors as a naval officer. Chris too was laid to rest amid the sound of bullets, buried with honors as a law-enforcement officer. I wish my mom could be honored in this way as well. You see, she was the woman behind these two men. She was, and is, the woman behind me. It is the nobleness of my family that I have dwelt on this past week as I am left to carry on.

My mom was sugar and spice and everything…firecrackers. She was kind and sweet, but look out if you crossed swords with her. Today I want to share nine of the things I told her last Sunday, and I hope that at least one stays in your brain so that my mom can have a lasting effect on you too. I picked an example to go along with each, and I hope you will feel free to laugh. I laughed as I wrote this.

1.   Don't run from a necessary fight.

One evening when Chris was fourteen and I was ten, Mom was cooking dinner, and Dad was having his customary glass of wine. We saw Chris speeding across the lawn, headed for the front door. A neighborhood bully was close behind, and it wasn't the first time. I think Chris always thought that what happened next was my dad's doing. But in reality, it was my mom who said in her soft Southern accent, "Dick, not this time. He can't keep running."

My dad met my brother at the door and said, "Stand your ground."

I remember screaming something like, "Chris is going to die, and it's your fault!" But he survived, and he never ran away from another fight.

2.   Influence people by asking questions instead of telling them what to do.

My friends who work with me will understand this. The reason that I say things like, "John, are you sure you want to damage that relationship by sending that e-mail?" is because I first heard my mother say, "Dick, are you sure you want to wear that red shirt with those green plaid pants?" My mom was able to influence people without telling them what to do.

3.   Be kind and help people in need.

About a year ago, Mom and I were getting her nails done. As I paid, I saw her looking into the mirror. She would smile and nod to the person she saw. I realized that she didn't recognize her reflection. She walked up to me and said, "Julie, there's an old woman over there. Go over and invite her to dinner with us." I tried not to laugh, and I gently pointed out that we were the only ones left in the shop. Mom was furious and said, "If you hadn't taken your own damn time, she'd be having dinner with us right now." I learned over these years with my mom and other elderly people at CARE-Assist that we become more of what we were when we were young. The cranky people get crankier and the sweet people, like Mom, get sweeter. Disease could not shake a kind heart.

4.   Be a patriot.

My dad loved serving his country and did it with passion. But Mom always made it clear that she was just as much in the military as he was.

When I was little, we went to movies at the military base because it was cheaper. Before the shows everyone stood as they played the national anthem. One night, the national anthem came on. A flag waved on the screen. And no one stood. Except my parents. I was old enough to think that being one of only three people standing in a full movie theater was not a very attractive thing to do. So I sat. But not for long, because my mom on one side and my dad on the other jerked me up by the collar and shoulder. Mom hissed at me, "Don't you ever sit down for this country." My father turned to stare at the audience, and many stood. I was embarrassed that day but never again. I was very aware of the sacrifice people had made on my behalf. For this reason, the flag flies at my house every day.

5.   Appreciate the good things in life, up to a point.

My parents were not extravagant people, but years ago they purchased a set of Waterford crystal. Mom loved it and we used it often, but we all held our breath with each use because no one wanted to be the first to break a glass or goblet. When Chris was seventeen, we came home one Saturday night and found him having a glass of wine with a date in the den. Mom was horrified and once again sent my dad to do the dirty work. When he came back, Chris and his date were still finishing their glasses of wine but using the cheap wine glasses, not the Waterford. It was a different time.

However, I think I can count on one hand the number of times in my life that we used the silver. That's because it took too long to polish it, and there were always more important things to do. Mom had a little sign in her window that said, "An immaculate house is the sign of a misspent life."

6.   Laugh.

I come from a funny family. Mom. Dad. Chris. Me. We all laughed. At ourselves and at each other. Let me give you a few examples. Mom was a teacher in the early years and read the paper every day. She was educated and loved to learn. But somehow she made it into her for-ties with a vocabulary flaw. She was reading an article to my dad, as she would frequently do, and said that "someone had 'myzled' someone else."

My dad looked at her quizzically and said, "What?"

Mom said, "Myzled."

Dad leaned over to look at the word and said, "That's misled! You haven't realized that before now?" We laughed about it for many years.

I'm the second kid. As my nephew, Rick, knows, it's hard to be the second kid. Chris had a perfectly complete baby book. Only my name was in mine. My mom's dresser drawer was full of things Chris had made, but there were few trinkets from me. I always kidded mom about this, and I was especially hard on her for having one of Chris's baby shoes bronzed but not one of mine. When I came home from college at Thanksgiving my freshman year, Mom excitedly brought me upstairs.

"Guess what?" she said with a twinkle in her eye. "I had Chris's other baby shoe bronzed." She loved the look on my face as I processed this and then burst out laughing as she explained that it really was my baby shoe and she was making up for the whole baby-book issue.

Mom never could remember that it was Gladys Knight, not Gladys Pipps.

I remember coming down for breakfast one April Fool's Day and there were Styrofoam peanuts in our cereal bowls.

My aunt Gloria says that Mom laughed as she talked, and I know that I do that too.

7. Be practical when talking to kids.

Like many moms, mine told me that I could be anything I wanted to be. But when I said I wanted to be an astronaut or a veterinarian, she'd say something like, "Well, not that. You aren't good enough at science for that."

I'd say, "You said I could be anything I wanted to be."

And she would say, "Okay, there are exceptions." But she was right. She knew me and my limitations, as well as my potential.

I want to share with you why I never experimented with drugs. You parents may want to use this technique. Mom took me aside one day when I was little and drugs were rampant, and she said, "If you were ever to have a baby before you get married, I would still love you just as much." Now, this kind of worried me because I didn't know at that time exactly where babies came from. But then she said the most important part. "But if you ever got hooked on drugs, I wouldn't be able to take it. I can't bear to see a child of mine die that way. So I have decided that if that happens, I will just kill you myself."

8.   Be mysterious.

After Mom moved back to Virginia, we had many loose photos that had adorned the walls of their home in San Diego. I gave her the idea of combining them and making books, and the result was two beautiful albums that spanned the decades. But Mom had a surprise. She had kept, for all those years, a picture of a man named Don who'd asked her to marry him about the same time Dad asked. She chose Dad, of course, and history unfolded. But when she made the books, she decided to give Don a page. I still remember Chris's reaction: "Who is that?" he said.

I said, "He's the guy who was almost our dad!"

Chris said, "Well, get him out of there!"

I said, "It's Mom's album, and anyway, I have the necklace he gave her." I'm not sure Chris ever fully recovered from the shock.

9.   Be a good stranger.

I actually didn't learn this one from Mom—I learned it through Mom. One day I was waiting for something urgent in the mail. I was already stretched and in a state of "perpetual behindedness" at home. As I reached in the mailbox, all that was there was a note saying that my mail had been held because the box had gotten too full and that I couldn't claim it for two days. But whatever it was, I needed it that day. I tearfully called the post office and begged a man named Claude to send someone out. When he said no, I blurted out my whole story. He sighed in frustration and said, "Give me ten minutes." I was expecting a call, but instead there was a knock at the door. The man standing there was holding a big pile of mail—my mail—and said, "Claude sent me. Is there anything I can help you with while I'm here?" I can't explain it, but I knew he meant it. As though I could have asked him to help me with anything and he would have done it. Similarly, the Giant ladies—who are not large people but who work at the Giant grocery store—hug me every visit and ask how Mom is. Women I didn't know would frequently come up to me when we were out, put a hand on my shoulder, and say wisely, "Appreciate these times." And many of you know how the red carpet gets rolled out for the Nielsen women at local restaurants. The friends who stuck it out were critically important, but strangers were special.

So I hope that these nine items are memorable. Erica and Rick, I especially hope they shape you the way they shaped me. Because of my mom, I'll invest well in people and invest my money well too. I'll have an organized house so I can fool people into thinking it's clean. My hair will almost always look good when I go out. And when I look at myself in the mirror, I'll make sure to see the things I'd rather not see. I will make sure the color of my carpet matches the color of my pets. And oh yes—I will eat out.

As I close, I want to share one more thing with you. Many of you might not know it, but I developed arthritis in my early twenties. Until about forty,

I really struggled with it—frequently at night, hardly able to move. I sometimes felt like I could not be any more alone. When my dad died at a young age, and I too was at a young age, I thought I would never recover. And I frequently felt so alone. When I got the call from an old family friend that Mom's problems were not just age, I was confronted with my worst nightmare. I felt so alone. Not too long after Chris died, as I was handling his affairs, I ended up in a roadside motel outside of Roanoke because the big-name hotels were booked. I was scared and so sad. Sitting on the bed at two in the morning, I never felt more alone. And over the last four years, there were so many nights where I would sit in my living room before falling into bed, and I'd hear only the clock. And I never felt so alone.

But in each of those circumstances, I have always been able to look back and see that I wasn't truly alone. God's hand was always present. And I could look back and see how the circumstances were all linked, and how things were resolved in ways I never would have imagined. People are very well aware that I haven't just lost my mom, that I have lost my immediate family. But His faithfulness continues, and I am alive and well because of it.

I read Condoleezza Rice's book *Extraordinary, Ordinary People: A Memoir of My Family* last year, and I made note of the last paragraph of the book. It changed how I look at my family as I stand before you today. She wrote, "It has been their presence, not their absence, that I've experienced. 'You are well prepared for whatever is ahead of you,' I could hear them say. 'Now don't forget that you are God's child and He will keep you in His care.' They remain by my side. And I feel today, as before, the overwhelming and unconditional love of the extraordinary, ordinary parents that I was so blessed to have."

My mom is my hero. Strong and wise. And I hope you see her in me. So tonight at five, I hope everyone will come to my house for a glass of wine, and we will toast my mom. We'll be using the Waterford, but don't look for the silver. And before you go to bed tonight, please call your mother.

Listen to Martina McBride's song "In My Daughter's Eyes," and it will complete the picture I painted that day. My friend sang it at the funeral. One of the most moving things for me at the funeral was the number of hospice employees and employees from the replacement caregiving company who came. People who'd spent only a day with Mom were there. I was touched, especially by Maria's hug before she left. "I knew you meant it," I said to her through tears. The CARE-Home employees who had been with us so long were nowhere to be found. But my friends and supporters showed up in force.

In a way, it was so different. And in a way, it was just as awful. Dad's death had been painfully swift. Although his health wasn't great, we weren't expecting it. The pain of that phone call from Chris was piercing and lives in my memory. Chris's death was even more painful. We aren't supposed to lose siblings, especially not before we lose our parents. That phone call from Kim haunts me. Secretly, I think I have posttraumatic stress disorder. Those calls and words come back to me when I lose the battle with sadness. But Mom was different. In reality, she died over eight years, zooming to an end after the assault at the hands of her caregiver. Even that day, I was different—better emotionally than two months after Chris died. I showered and felt oddly put together. I played the events of the last month over and over in my brain. I lost the ability to touch her and hold her hand that day, but I had already lost most of her along the way. I hadn't been able to ask for her thoughts or opinions for two years. Our conversations had been pretend conversations, with me holding up both ends, letting Mom feel like she was having a real conversation. I'd been prepared.

And I was haunted by Grace. The official charge was "assault on an incapacitated adult." The official cause of Mom's death was stroke, although no doctor ever examined her for that. But as the days roll on, I think about whether we let my mom down. She had been assaulted, and she never recovered. And it quietly went down in the legal system as a misdemeanor. Or maybe the reason didn't matter by then. For weeks after the assault, I would faithfully check the weekly crime section in the paper, hoping to at least see it mentioned—some indicator to the world that there was danger to the elderly. But there was nothing. I would have to direct attention to the danger, or it wasn't going to happen.

Two days after Mom died, I went to the gym. The gym routine had meant so much during the time I cared for Mom. The mental benefits of fitness are, in my mind, huge. Stay active. The gym hummed with activity, and life went on around me. I felt the way I had felt in the airport all those years ago. No one could see what was going on in my life. That was another lesson for me—remember as we interact with people, those we know as well as strangers, that we don't know what they are dealing with right now. And be kind.

My friends Rick and Miriam gave me another one of those amazing gifts. They flew in right away and were at the funeral. Miriam and I spent hours sorting through items still left at the condo, making a pile for me, a pile for the kids, and a pile for donation. Later, after the kids picked up what was special to them, Miriam and Rick were at the condo without me when a truck showed up to pick up the donations, leaving empty rooms that held nothing for me.

Mom and I both had peace now, and I could feel the next chapter of my life opening up. But it would open only a crack before reality pulled me back.

CHAPTER 20

Deception

"One daughter, two criminals," I thought, sitting in the courtroom next to Pat. That is one of the most important takeaways of this book. In other words, don't live in a dream world and think that people are not trying to get money or otherwise injure the people you love. Don't get me wrong—I'm not so jaded as to think that it's everyone. But we have to be smart and realize that even one is one criminal too many. They are out there, and they might not look like monsters.

We saw Detective Mullins and greeted him. The world of the court revolved around us—sad cases of people who messed up frequently and silly cases of people who had tripped and run afoul of the law and weren't the type to be there. And people like us—witnesses from another world. You see another side of life when you sit in a courtroom. Barring the fact that my mother was dead and I was there to see someone I'd thought I loved get convicted of assaulting her, it all seemed oddly normal. It was September 25—not even a month since Mom died.

Looking at the opposite side of the courtroom, I noticed an older woman and man. "Maybe that's Grace's sister," I said to Pat.

"Maybe," Pat noted. And then we noticed the agitation. The detective looked surprised. He was talking to the prosecutor, who also looked surprised. They both turned to look at us.

"I think they are looking at us," I said flatly.

"Something is wrong," Pat said. "Here he comes."

The detective was walking toward us, and I braced myself for news. "I don't want you to stand up, and I don't want you to make a scene."

"Okay," I thought, "why does he think I'm going to make a scene?"

"Do you know that woman sitting over there?" he asked me.

I turned to look at the woman Pat and I had studied earlier. "No, I don't, but it might be Grace's sister."

"Julie," the detective said, looking very concerned, "*that is Grace.*"

CHAPTER 21

Looking for Monsters

t hadn't registered at first. I was stunned. The person I'd thought was Grace wasn't Grace. The person CARE-Home had provided as Grace was not Grace. Shock turned into anger—or maybe fury. I had gone to them to avoid this. My final decision on caregiving had been based on having a company do the footwork to conduct background and reference checks. I had gone to them thinking that I wasn't equipped to root out untrained people and potential criminals. After running Mom's bank account dangerously low by paying their premium rates, I now knew that they had not been equipped either. And they didn't know who they had employed or who they had sent to my mother's home. Regardless, we had been lied to for three years, my mother had been assaulted, and now she was dead.

The incident quickly turned into much more than the assault on my mom. Immigration issues and stolen identity came into play, and the investigation was turned over to a federal investigator, Brandon Creech, at the Department of Homeland Security (DHS). Grace, or whoever she was, had disappeared. And justice began to follow its slow and steady course.

Death didn't stop people from targeting Mom. I took a month-long sabbatical from work to write most of this book. As I was writing one day, I received a voice mail, clearly a holdover from taking all of Mom's calls for so many years. It was a man's voice—not providing any name or company name—telling me he was calling about the delivery of my "I've Fallen and I Can't Get Up" system. I hit the delete button. "Some scam," I thought. The next week, the same message. But with the third week and the third identical message, I'd had it. How many elderly people were these jokers calling? I dialed the number.

"Hello," a young man said. "Are you calling about your "I've Fallen and I Can't Get Up" system?"

"Yes, I am," I said softly, trying to sound like an elderly woman.

"Do you know how it works?" he asked.

"No, I don't believe I do." I said, playing along. He went on to describe it, asking me if I remembered the woman in the commercials from years back. "I don't think I could pay for that," I said, remembering that the message had said someone had paid for it.

"Oh, don't worry—the Virginia Department of Health paid for it for you, it says here."

I switched to my normal voice and said, "I don't think the Virginia Department of Health does that type of thing."

"Oh, that's because it's the *federal* Department of Health...that's it...the *federal* department."

"Hmm," I replied. "You and I both probably know there is no federal Department of Health, right?"

"Lady," he exclaimed, exasperated, "what do you want with me?"

"I'm just collecting information to share with the police," I said calmly.

"Oh, lady, I'm just trying to make a living. I'm hanging up now." He slammed down the phone. I hadn't played along enough to find out what his real objective was.

Although I laughed as I hung up the phone, I grew more concerned about how many people these people were calling. Most, I was quite confident, were a lot older than I was and not nearly as suspicious. "Write the book," I thought. "Focus on one objective."

But the following week, there was another call. This time, I happened to answer the phone. There was the same recording, and this time I was connected. "Press one to talk with an associate," I heard after the message. I pressed one, with no plan in mind. This time the man at the other end sounded older.

"Yes, you called me about some system?" I said in my elder voice when he answered.

"Yes, ma'am," he replied. "One of your kids paid for the system for you, and I'm just calling to arrange for delivery."

"Really?" I responded. "That seems strange." I didn't say why.

"Oh, wait," he said, fumbling audibly through papers, "maybe it was a friend who paid for it—I can't find my paper here with the name."

"How does it work?" I asked.

"Miss Julie, are we friends?" he asked.

"Why, I suppose so," I answered.

"Well, Miss Julie, it is very important that you accept delivery of this. How many times have you fallen in the last year and not been able to get up?"

"Well, not at all," I said, "but I worry about that."

I'm sure he thought he had a live one. "Well, since I'm your friend, I'm going to help make sure it doesn't happen ever, okay?"

"Okay," I said. "How does it work?"

"Well, we'll send you this system, and you just need to pay us $34.99 a month so we can monitor it for you. We just need your charge card. But because we're friends, if you don't like it, I'm going to let you return it, but we can still be friends."

I was about to get stuck. I didn't want to commit further without thinking about my alternatives, so I said, "I'll have to talk to my daughter about this."

"Well, okay," he said, "but if you tell me you are rejecting this, I'm going to have to call the person who bought it for you and let them know you are rejecting their gift."

"I'll talk to my daughter," I said again before hanging up.

Care Concept #12: Look for Monsters

People are in pursuit of the elderly. They may be attractive, kind, and trust-worthy-looking people. They may be strangers, and they may be people you know. Trust people when you choose to for your own life, but maintain a high level of vigilance when it comes to a loved one. Watch out for one or more of the following:

- Rip-offs (which are more minor and could consume smaller amounts of money)
- Financial fraud (which are more major and could consume critical savings)
- Theft (of money, valuables, or special items)
- Physical harm (periodic or ongoing abuse)

I could read the exasperation in the e-mail when I corresponded with one of the officers I knew. "Any ideas on what I could do about these guys?" I had asked. Being a crusader can wear other people out.

After doing some checking, he got back in touch and said, "Julie, you're going to have to just file a report with the police; we can't take this one on. Or maybe the Better Business Bureau."

I knew the police have too many calls and reports to handle something like this. So I took a break from writing to alert a local news outlet. I saw a small article in the paper weeks later about the scam and their activity in several states. The police can't stop the many criminals or the barely legal people who are targeting seniors—there are simply too many. But education can stop them. And *education* is the purpose of this book.

CHAPTER 22

Finding Grace (II)

Hurricane Sandy brushed Washington, DC, in October 2012 as it barreled up the coast. We had all made preparations in anticipation of a hit. But the brush was frightening enough for me. I huddled with the pets on the first floor in case a tree came crashing into the house. On the one hand, it was nice not to have to worry about anyone else, but on the other, I was oddly alone. I sat on the couch and watched the trees whip back and forth at unnerving angles.

The next day I went out with Sasha to see how the neighborhood had fared in the storm. I saw my long-time neighbor Mary. I had heard from other neighbors that she had been experiencing "issues." I had seen signs of trouble myself but nothing urgent—and I didn't see her much.

"I'm moving," she said flatly as Sasha and I crossed the street to say *hello*.

"Really, where to?" I asked.

She said, "I'm moving to a place called CARE-Assist, nearby."

That feeling of being in the right place at the right time washed over me. "I know it well, Mary—my mom used to live there, and you will love it," I replied. I immediately pictured the sunny sitting rooms and cheerful décor.

Mary brightened. "Will you come talk to my daughter with me?" she asked.

We walked to her house. As her daughter and I talked, I saw myself from years ago. She was single and didn't know what to do. "Please let me help," I said, and she promised she would.

"Will you come visit me, Julie?" Mary asked.

"Yes, I will. Very soon," I said as I got up to leave.

A few weeks later, Hailey joined me for a visit to CARE-Assist. She had made pet rocks to share with residents. Many of the same faces were still there. Surprisingly, staff members came out to offer their condolences. I wasn't expecting them to know Mom had died. And it was much the same as it had always been. "Hi, Peaches," our old friend said from his perch in the café. Mary was with him, and she looked content.

I kept Mom's ring locked away for a few months—it was the one I had taken from her at CARE-Assist and returned to her at the condo. But when I was ready, I took it out and had it resized for my right ring finger. It replaced my grandmother's first engagement ring, which I had worn since Mom gave it to me for high-school graduation. I beamed when I put it on, and the jewelry-store employees gathered around me to share the moment. They had resized it while I waited, out of deference to my brushes with crime that made me hesitant to leave the ring with anyone. When I came home, I got the rest of Mom's jewelry out to study it. My heart skipped a beat when I saw a small box with Mom's handwriting. It said "Grandbill's Ring" on the top. I opened it and found Grandbill's other ring—one not stolen at CARE-Assist. I hadn't realized there was a second one. It's now on my left hand. It is probably her wedding band, but it has a distinctly modern look. Many times during each day, I look down and see my parents on my right hand and my grandparents on my left. I get a similar feeling when I go to the shooting range and fire Chris's gun, and even more so when I hit the bull's-eye.

This is where our story felt like it was *supposed* to end, with me finding my footing in a new world, with me finding my own grace. But it refused to, and so the book had to wait. It would sit, with me tweaking it periodically, for over three years, while the story wound its way to its conclusion. I actually would have made it stop and let the book get published. But it wasn't up to me. The federal investigation needed to be protected, and I complied (although not always patiently) with the official request to delay.

CHAPTER 23

Finding Grace (III)

t was February 23, 2015, and the call was anticlimactic. I was rushing out the door with Sadie.

Sasha died in late 2014, and I had added Sadie to the family shortly afterward. I almost didn't take her from the rescue facility in DC. I knew I could not handle a puppy. They were telling me she was two, but I could tell she was young. But sitting alone with her in the backyard of the building, she bounded over, put her head in my lap, and looked at me with soulful puppy eyes and a wrinkled brow. "You look like you need a family," I said to her, "and so do I." She seemed to understand, and suddenly I was looking at her in my rearview mirror as we drove home. I would find out quickly why she ended up needing to be rescued (after she ate through a windowsill, three pieces of molding, four pillows, and too many "indestructible" dog toys to count), but she would later turn into the ideal companion after professional training and some doggy maturity. It struck me soon after getting Sadie that I hadn't been laughing much. Don't get me wrong; I was happy again in general. I just wasn't laughing. Now she and her antics make me laugh every day.

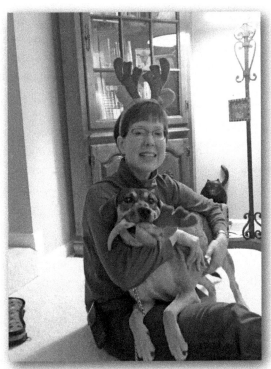

Trying to get Sadie to cooperate for a Christmas-card photo. Laughter is good.

The phone was ringing. I glanced at the number, planning on ignoring the call, but it was Brandon from DHS. Every few weeks I would call to see if he had any updates. There was never much he could share other than that the investigation was moving along, but he was patient with me and told me what he could. Each time, he'd end with, "Okay, I'll call you when I have something more to tell you," and I'd say, "Okay... talk to you in a few weeks." I had been hopeful early on, after testifying in front of a federal grand jury just a few months after Mom died. But then there was mounting evidence and lots of endless research and investigations. I was scared to death of our case getting lost. And until I could publicize what happened, I was failing—failing to make anything good come out of what had happened. I was desperate to do that, and the waiting was excruciating.

The woman I knew as Grace was really named Hilda. I still refer to her as "Fake Grace" because it's hard to call her by a new name. And she disappeared the day she left my mom's condo. For months that stretched into years, her family was adamant that they hadn't seen her—a rather difficult tale to believe, in my opinion as well as law enforcement's. A top detective in Fairfax County who worked closely with the federal government had gotten involved. Everyone involved tried diligently to find her. Meanwhile, the investigation grew and grew. Multiple federal agencies would become involved, and the subpoenas and potential charges began to pile up.

Later I would learn that it wasn't all about Hilda. There was Grace—the real Grace, Hilda's sister—her husband, Emmanuel, and another family member. They easily slid Hilda by CARE-Home, substituting one for the other. I had believed the promise that CARE-Home was more capable than I was to hire and manage the right caregiver. The ease with which the family did it still surprises (and angers) me.

The government has two solid ways of preventing crimes like this. The easiest is the I-9 form that employers complete on every new employee to verify identity and eligibility to work in the United States. I'll never understand why all of the elderly people in the care of CARE-Home caregivers weren't important enough for a thorough check. Did CARE-Home rush? Did they even look? The check is so simple, and I have done hundreds in my career (and thousands indirectly). There was a familial resemblance between Hilda and Grace, but the two women were like night and day. Hilda is a very large woman—tall and big, like a mountain. Grace is much shorter and smaller, and older. It would be difficult to confuse the two. Plus, Hilda had said she didn't drive, but she'd provided a driver's license (her sister's) for the I-9.

The second way to check someone's identity is through E-Verify. Although not yet required of all employers, it's an excellent way of confirming who you are really talking to. At the end of the process, the system offers a picture of anyone with immigrant status to confirm the applicant you are looking at is who she says she is. It should be federally required, in my opinion, at least for all caregiving companies and assisted-living facilities, as it is for government contractors. The Commonwealth of Virginia, where I live, does not require it. There is no way around the fact that our most precious citizens are frequently cared for by immigrants because of the low wages; the potential for abuse is obvious.

There were attempted sham marriages and all sorts of efforts to keep Hilda off the government's radar. For someone like me who values our country so much, it was frustrating to see this family so flagrantly break our laws. And now the incidents of poor training came back to haunt me. What I had classified as individual slipups were really a pattern of poor care—from the firm I had been told was the best. I could only imagine how the less highly regarded companies might be screening and managing their employees. And of course, there was fraud and all sorts of contractual issues, since the company had erred in a big way.

"You're the only one I'd interrupt the dog walk for," I said as I answered the phone that February evening.

"You know I'd never be calling you this time of day if something hadn't happened," he replied. "We found Fake Grace."

I'm not sure how I was supposed to feel. I was elated at first. Brandon was pumped too, and he told me the story of how she was captured. The Friday before, she had made a reservation to fly to Ghana from JFK in New York. I wonder if she thought no one would be looking for her there. But they were watching for her, and up she popped on the federal radar. Then bad weather canceled the flight. Federal agents waited. And there she was again. She rebooked, and this time the weather was good. Federal agents met her at the gate. I learned that scaring people into trying to leave the country is a good way to catch them. I also learned that there are jails at international airports. "Julie, people like you have no clue about things like this," Brandon had said, laughing.

Hilda was booked in New York and was soon extradited to Fairfax County. I pulled her up online and saw five felonies listed—quite different from the one misdemeanor I was familiar with. "One day soon, I will be able to sit down and tell you everything," Brandon promised that night before hanging up. I told him how proud I was of everyone involved—and him in particular. Later, a friend would text and say congratulations, but celebrating didn't feel quite right. Hilda had played a big role in my family, and picturing anyone I know in jail was unpleasant.

I wanted so much to ask Hilda and the family, "Are you happy? Was it worth it?" We all lost. My life is forever changed. When others watch the video of the assault, they don't hear sound. But I do. Hilda's screaming is stuck in my head—no matter how I try to erase it. So is the expression on Mom's face as Hailey and I walked in—it is etched there in my memory. And Grace and Hilda's family...I'm sure it is now destroyed, torn by jail, impending deportations, and accusations of blame.

Back to court I went, first in Fairfax County and then to federal court in Alexandria. I would see Hilda plead guilty and be sentenced in Fairfax. She served six months there and was then transferred to federal jail. Then there was a court visit to see Hilda plead in federal court, followed by one to see Grace plead. Then it was back again to see Hilda sentenced and then one to see Grace get sentenced. As I spoke in court at each sentencing, I was painfully aware that no sentence would fix what happened. But the message at each would—so each time, I asked the judge to send a message that abusing the elderly or putting them at risk is not okay. The judge in Fairfax in particular sent a powerful message as he sentenced Hilda. I was thrilled that the courtroom was packed. If one potential abuser heard, maybe he or she would think twice. And a lot of people who are or will become old heard about the risks we will all face.

A stranger—a woman who said she was a social worker and was assisting Hilda—caught me after Hilda's federal sentencing. I still don't know exactly who she was or how they met. She accidentally spoke in court after I did, before the judge realized she was out of place and had her sit down. But she seemed to indeed have been talking to Hilda. "Hilda loved your mom, and she loves you too," she said.

I didn't say much then, but deep down, I believed her. "Why did she do it?" I asked.

"She doesn't know," the stranger said. "Something she can't explain came over her. But she wants you to know it only happened once. And," she went on in a serious tone, "the blood on the sheets was from bloody noses." I wanted so badly to believe her, and I think I did.

CHAPTER 24

Lessons and the Real Ending, November 4, 2016

had to get up early each time I went to court. Traffic on Washington's Beltway is hard to call, so I would leave plenty of time. And today's visit was special—it was my last one. It was sentencing day for Emmanuel, Grace's husband. He had been involved in the whole plot as well. Today would usher in my time to talk and to finish this book.

Sadie and I walked in the early-morning darkness, and I thought about all that had transpired since Mom died. It was a crystal-clear morning, and the stars were out. I always feel close to Mom, Dad, and Chris on clear nights. As though they are just barely out of reach.

As I was leaving, I printed one of my favorite pictures of Mom and me and stuck it in my purse. Both of us were smiling for the camera, sitting at breakfast at the Ritz Carlton.

A lot had happened since Mom died. I decided to make a job change—a difficult decision to leave the friends who had seen me through so much. But a fresh start seemed to make sense. I felt like I had changed too. I had gone from a victim to an observer and now a plotter. I plotted how I would make sure at least one person's life was changed as a result of our story.

Not surprisingly, there had been attorneys, along with all the law-enforcement professionals. An attorney-friend had said early on, "Everyone else is represented...I think you should be too." So I identified someone with a background in elder abuse.

I laughed silently to myself one day as the CARE-Home attorney tried to bully me. I wanted to say, "Girl, you clearly don't realize all I've been through because *nothing* you can say or do is going to scare me." Instead I stared at her in cool silence and allowed her to finish. CARE-Home and I would reach an amicable agreement on the whole matter. And in the end, after disappearing the day everything unraveled, the owner of CARE-Home, would apologize. It was heartfelt, and despite the delay, it meant a lot. I figured that their attorney had said quickly after my call that day, "Don't talk to her—stay away." I thought of all the people they had cared for, and I believed that what happened was a result of carelessness, not intent. A larger company took them over, and I wondered if our incident was the driver behind the sale.

It was getting cold sitting in my car. I got the photo out and wrote a note to Brandon on the back, thanking him for all he had done. He had lived our case. And he cared so much. No one other than me cared that much. Now I was sitting next to him at the back of the courtroom. Emmanuel was on the other side of the room, a couple of rows up. I pulled the photo out and gave it to Brandon. "Now don't lose this," I said, noticing he didn't have anything with him to put it in.

"I won't. It means a lot," he said after reading the note. As another case was called and we all waited, Emmanuel looked over at me repeatedly, seeming to study me. I studied him back. What was in his face? Was it sadness at what had happened to my mom? Was it anger that I had stumbled onto their scheme and brought the whole thing down? Did they blame me, or did they regret what they had done? Hilda and Grace had avoided looking at me during our times in court. I tried hard, but I couldn't read his face.

It was over quickly, just like the other visits. Although he had pleaded guilty to the most serious of all the felonies, he was sentenced only to probation. You see, Emmanuel was now seventy-two. Hilda had gotten the worst of it—that was clear. Grace—sentenced to home confinement for a year, except for work—was the next worst off. Hilda was already deported. Emmanuel would be next. I suspected that Grace, although not deported, would also leave for Ghana before long.

Lessons

If you'd asked me early on in this odyssey, I would have given specific recommendations on what to do with regard to elder care. But looking back now, I won't. There are really five clear lessons.

1. Make a plan. Because when trouble arrives—and it will—there will be a plan. Regardless of resources, something will happen, and you will do something as a result of it. So we might as well create a plan earlier instead of later. I've had people say to me, "I have no money and no options," as though that means they can't have a plan. Don't wait for a catastrophe to figure out what to do.

2. Make an informed decision. You can do this for your parents or other family members or for yourself. Especially if you plan ahead—back to #1. Any decision we make regarding care for our loved ones or ourselves has inherent risk. Every single option. That is the depressing news. The encouraging news is that we can equip ourselves. Technology takes us to another level and increases our ability, with or without deep resources, to protect.

3. Never—never—let your guard down. The number of criminals isn't going to decrease. The elderly will always make rich targets. Law enforcement can go after them once something happens. But then it's too late. I wrote this book so that you can get ahead of crime—and hopefully avoid it.

4. Know that people are good at hiding things. Your parents and other older people in your life are often worse than you realize. If your dad is suddenly forgetting things, it's probably just sudden to you. This means that you'd better move fast.

5. Get the car. When you catch yourself saying that your frail or forgetful parent is still a good driver, get over it. Realize that frail and forgetful are both disqualifiers. I have triggered "the car reaction" in many people's plans by repeating what the CARE-Home nurse had said: "What if she [he] backs over a mother and a baby stroller?" I hit the mark every time, as the nurse did with me. We have to think about other people and the effect compromised driving could have on their lives.

I asked Brandon what advice he would share with readers in light of his law-enforcement view into crimes against seniors, and he shared six recommendations of his own:

1. Shop around for the right caregiver. When looking into a company, check the Better Business Bureau and look at complaints. Find out what their application process is. Specifically look at how they confirm someone's identity, background, eligibility, and so forth.

2. Once you choose a caregiving company and they have provided you with a caregiver of your choice, get to know that person. You have more leeway than the employer does and will learn a lot about education, life experiences, and immigration status.

3. Once you feel comfortable with your caregiver, it is time to set up the house. Nanny cams are great resources. You can use one or several. Leave items of value out at certain times and monitor them. If the person is trustworthy, items of value will not turn up missing.

4. Get to know your neighbors. Invite them to help with spot checks, and make sure they know you want to hear from them. They may hear or see something out of place.

5. Check your loved one for cuts and bruises. Unexplained injuries are an indicator that something is not right. Document injuries and have the caregiver explain what happened. "I don't know" is not acceptable.

6. Remember this is *your* loved one, and it is *your* right to make sure they are being cared for properly. There are no stupid questions for you to ask, or dumb ideas for you to use to protect them.

We were in the condo for roughly two years, at CARE-Assist for two years, and then back in the condo for over three with CARE-Home helping us. Since the assault, I have had many people say things to me like, "I'm so glad we love our caregiver."

"So did I." Then I sigh. "So did I." My job protecting my mother is done. Unfortunately, in the end, I didn't protect her the way I wanted to, but I think I did my best. However, my job protecting *your* parents is not done yet, so I will write, speak, and share about what I learned via every channel I can find. Because nothing is more important.

I told the judges in court that I needed to do just one thing. Specifically, I said, "That one thing is making sure that something good comes out of what happened. That one thing is making sure that I shine the brightest light possible on the dangers our frailest and most vulnerable citizens face at the hands of criminal, careless, and predatory people. And hopefully I will do something to change the trajectory of this crisis."

I have a daydream sometimes that Hilda will get in touch from Ghana and tell me what really happened. But regardless, I forgave her. I had to—not just because of my faith, but because I didn't want to stay stuck in time or let anger damage me physically or emotionally. Plus, I needed to move on with my life.

And now I'm off to do that one thing. When it's my turn to be one of those faces on the wall, I hope a lot of people are better off because I did.

About the Author

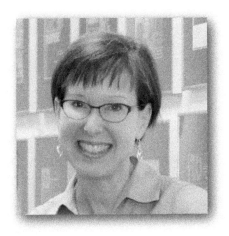

Julie Nielsen holds a degree in business administration from Auburn University and a graduate degree in human resources from Marymount University. She spent many years working long hours in leadership roles at various organizations in Northern Virginia, finding and managing talent, speaking about success in the work world, and coaching individuals on careers and job success.

Her life changed forever when her mother was diagnosed with Alzheimer's. She maintained detailed notes throughout her time caring for her mother because she knew there were lessons in her story that had to be shared.

Nielsen lives in the suburbs of Washington, DC, where she works as a business executive.

CPSIA information can be obtained
at www.ICGtesting.com
Printed in the USA
LVHW051457181020
669077LV00013B/2815